Calcium Urolithiasis

Pathogenesis, Diagnosis, and Management

TOPICS IN BONE AND MINERAL DISORDERS

Series Editor: **Louis V. Avioli, M.D.**
Washington University School of Medicine
St. Louis, Missouri

PAGET'S DISEASE OF BONE
Frederick R. Singer, M.D.

THE BONE BIOPSY
Jenifer Jowsey, D. Phil.

CALCIUM UROLITHIASIS: Pathogenesis, Diagnosis,
and Management
Charles Y.C. Pak, M.D.

A Continuation Order Plan is available for this series. A continuation order will bring delivery of each new volume immediately upon publication. Volumes are billed only upon actual shipment. For further information please contact the publisher.

Calcium Urolithiasis

Pathogenesis, Diagnosis, and Management

Charles Y. C. Pak, M.D.
The University of Texas Health Science Center at Dallas

PLENUM MEDICAL BOOK COMPANY
New York and London

Library of Congress Cataloging in Publication Data

Pak, Charles Y
  Calcium urolithiasis.

  (Topics in bone and mineral disorders)
  Includes bibliographical references and index.
  1. Calculi, Urinary. 2. Calcium metabolism disorders. I. Title. II. Series. [DNLM: 1.
Urinary calculi. WJ100.3 P152c]
RC916.P34   616.6'22   78-4083
ISBN 978-1-4684-2453-9   ISBN 978-1-4684-2451-5 (eBook)
DOI 10.1007/978-1-4684-2451-5

© 1978 Plenum Publishing Corporation
Softcover reprint of the hardcover 1st edition 1978
227 West 17th Street, New York, N. Y. 10011

Plenum Medical Book Company is an imprint of Plenum Publishing Corporation

Foreword

"People . . . see you sweat in agony, turn pale, turn red, tremble, vomit your very blood, suffer strange contractions and convulsions, sometimes shed great tears from your eyes, discharge thick, black and frightful urine, or have it stopped up by some sharp rough stone that cruelly pricks and flays the neck of your penis."* These 16th century frustrations of Michel de Montaigne which most graphically reflect his experience with renal colic still plague approximately 1 per 1000 individuals in the United States annually. Since as many as 75% of clinically-apparent episodes of renal colic represent single nonrecurring events, physicians not infrequently approach the differential diagnosis of nephrolithiasis in a less than adequate fashion and assume that the incident may probably never recur after the single attack. However, the ureteral or bladder stone actually represents one form of abnormal crystalline precipitation; parenchymal nephrocalcinosis, silently progressive azotemia, and asymptomatic renal pelvic calculi may also stem from the same pathological process(es) which conditioned the formation of the ureteral or bladder stone. In this regard it is worth emphasizing that the postmortem incidence of renal calculi is some tenfold greater than that presumed from surveys wherein a clinical attack of nephrolithiasis is the sole determinant.

*In *Familiar Medical Quotations*. M. B. Strauss, Ed. Little Brown, Boston, 1968, p. 646.

The last decade has witnessed the birth of new knowledge in urolithiasis research. More sophisticated testing parameters which help discriminate stone formers from non-stone-formers have been established, and certain rigid diagnostic criteria have been defined for patients with calcium urolithiasis and hypercalciuria. In this monograph, Dr. Pak not only reviews current concepts regarding physicochemical and biochemical factors which normally prevent crystalloid deposition within the kidney but also presents a most coherent and lucid description of the many pathological insults which initiate and perpetuate calculous disease in humans.

Montaigne, who, when plagued with renal colic "never found three doctors of the same opinion,"* would have obtained enormous benefit from the last chapter, which outlines some practical guidelines for the diagnosis and management of calcium urolithiasis. Although in modern times the many managerial discrepancies among physicians caring for patients with renal colic have been refined, there is still a demanding need for practical and therapeutic guidelines. Dr. Pak's refreshing monograph, which actually represents a summation of his vast experience in the field, should serve the frustrated physician and patient with colic quite well.

Louis V. Avioli, M.D.
Shoenberg Professor of Medicine

St. Louis

---

*de Montaigne, M. *The Autobiography of Michel de Montaigne*. M. Lowenthal, Ed. Random House, New York, p. 212.

Preface

There has been an explosion of research activity and an increasing public awareness concerning urolithiasis during the past decade. Considerable information is already available regarding the cause, diagnosis, and management of renal stones. Unfortunately, however, this information is often confined to specialists and is not generally available to the practicing physician. The author was therefore asked to summarize the current status of the urolithiasis field, from the perspectives of both pathogenesis and management.

In undertaking the writing of this volume, the author has tried to maintain objectivity, and has provided different points of view whenever possible. He acknowledges, however, that his conclusions may have been influenced by his personal experiences and research endeavor. He is also fully aware that continued progress in urolithiasis research will undoubtedly require reexamination of many of the hypotheses and conclusions presented herein. It is his hope that this text will provide a suitable background for making such an assessment.

The author would like to thank Cheryl Northcutt for editorial assistance, Linda Brinkley and Judith Townsend for their guidance in the preparation of Chapter 7, and Linda Higgins for clerical assistance.

Charles Y. C. Pak

Contents

Chapter 1

Introduction

During the past decade, rapid progress has been made in urolithiasis research. This advancement has encompassed four approaches: physical chemistry and biochemistry, physiology, mechanism of drug action, and diagnosis and management (Figure 1). The first approach seeks to isolate the specific physicochemical and biochemical properties of the urinary environment that predispose to formation of renal stones. The second approach focuses on physiological derangements or metabolic defects that might be etiologically important in stone formation. In other words, these two approaches address the causes of renal-stone formation *in vitro* and *in vivo*; specifically, they inquire into the nature of "stone-forming" urine and the reasons that certain patients are prone to form renal stones.

Biochemical and physiological advances have opened the way for research into the mechanism of drug action. The study of *in vitro* and *in vivo* effects of various therapeutic modalities is gradually making it possible to ascertain whether these modalities "reverse" physiological derangements and physicochemical abnormalities in the urine of patients with urolithiasis.

The last approach deals with improved diagnosis and management of urolithiasis. The development of diagnostic criteria for various causes of urolithiasis evolved naturally from a better understanding of the underlying physiological derangements associated with stone formation. These advances have made it possi-

1

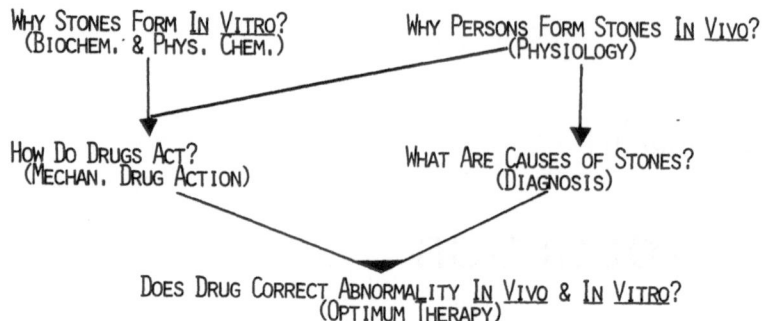

FIGURE 1. Four approaches in urolithiasis research.

ble to begin the formulation of a scheme for rational therapy of urolithiasis whereby a specific treatment may be chosen for each cause of stone formation. The regimen so chosen is presumably best able to correct the abnormality *in vivo* and *vitro*, i.e., to restore normal physicochemical urinary environment and physiologic function.

This book summarizes advances achieved by these four approaches that are relevant to renal stones containing calcium. Such calcareous renal stones can be categorized on the basis of principal abnormality—hypercalciuria, hyperuricosuria, or hyperoxaluria (Table I). Each category will be discussed separately from the perspective of all four approaches of urolithiasis research.

TABLE I. Classification of Calcium Urolithiasis

I. Hypercalciuria	II. Hyperuricosuria
1. Absorptive hypercalciuria	1. Primary
a. Type I	2. Dietary
b. Type II	III. Hyperoxaluria
c. Type III (hypophosphatemic)	1. Primary
2. Renal hypercalciuria	2. Enteric
3. Primary hyperparathyroidism	

Chapter 2 reviews physicochemical and biochemical requirements for stone formation in urine and discusses the role of inhibitors and promoters. It describes various techniques for the quantitation of the crystallization process—state of saturation, limit of metastability, crystal growth and aggregation, and heterogeneous nucleation. This review provides a basis for the understanding of stone formation and of the mechanism of drug action in the various disorders that are discussed in subsequent chapters.

Chapter 3 considers calcium urolithiasis associated with hypercalciuria. It discusses the role of hypercalciuria in stone formation as well as causes of hypercalciuria. Since intestinal hyperabsorption of calcium is frequently associated with hypercalciuria, this chapter also reviews possible pathogenetic mechanisms and the potential involvement of vitamin D metabolism. Next to be considered are the clinical presentation and diagnostic criteria for the two major forms of hypercalciuria, absorptive and renal hypercalciurias. Chapter 3 concludes with a discussion of the mode of action and indications for various treatment modalities, e.g., sodium cellulose phosphate, orthophosphate, and thiazide.

Chapter 4 is concerned with the third major form of hypercalciuria—hypercalciuria associated with hypercalcemia, particularly primary hyperparathyroidism. Since hypercalcemia may be considered a sequela of the loss of calcium homeostatic control, this chapter reviews various calcium homeostatic mechanisms, especially those involving hormonal regulation. The cause of renal-stone formation and the clinical presentation, diagnostic criteria, and management of primary hyperparathyroidism are discussed at some length. The condition of primary hyperparathyroidism is then contrasted with other causes of hypercalcemia.

Chapter 5 discusses calcium-stone formation associated with hyperuricosuria. The evidence supporting an important etiological role for monosodium urate is provided. The clinical presentation, diagnostic criteria, and management of this interesting disorder are then given.

Chapter 6 deals primarily with urolithiasis associated with enteric hyperoxaluria. The causes of stone formation and of hyperoxaluria are explored. This chapter then considers the mode of action

and indications for various therapeutic modalities for the hyperoxaluria.

It is apparent from the foregoing discussion that considerable
improvement has been made in the diagnosis and management of
patients with calcium urolithiasis. Unfortunately, however, delivery of these improvements in patient care is often restricted to specialized centers and is not yet available in the setting of the practicing physician. As an initial step toward making these
improvements more widely available, Chapter 7 provides practical
guidelines for the diagnosis and management of different causes of
calcium urolithiasis.

Chapter 2

Physical Chemistry
of Stone Formation

Major progress has been made during the past decade in the physical chemistry and biochemistry of stone formation. The development of improved techniques [1-5] for the quantitation of various processes of stone formation was crucial in this advancement. These techniques have begun to be used in delineating the factors that regulate stone formation and defining the physicochemical environment of urine that predisposes to formation of stones. They have also been applied to establishing the physicochemical action of various therapeutic regimens for nephrolithiasis [6-10] and to quantitating the response to treatment. [11,12]

SCHEME FOR STONE FORMATION

Before the advent of more sophisticated physicochemical approaches for the study of stone disease, three theories were invoked for the formation of stones: (1) The *precipitation-crystallization* [13,14] theory considered stone formation as a physicochemical process of precipitation of stone salts from a supersaturated urine. (2) In the *matrix* theory, [15-17] the crystal nidus was believed to develop in organic matrix, probably under the in-

5

fluence of the matrix, analogous to the formation of bone. (3) The
inhibitor theory [18-20] assumed that urine normally contains inhibitors of crystallization. The lack or absence of inhibitors in the
urine of stone-formers would permit development of stones.

These theories are not necessarily mutually exclusive. Irrespective of a particular theory proposed for stone formation, an es-
sential requirement is a state of supersaturation of urine with respect to constituents of stone. It is obvious that a crystal nidus
cannot be established either *de novo* or in an organic matrix from
urine that is undersaturated with respect to that nidus. Since the
inhibitors of nucleation prevent nucleation from a supersaturated
solution, their role in an undersaturated solution probably has no
significance in stone formation.

The current scheme for stone formation incorporates previous
theories as well as other factors—e.g., promoters of nucleation,
crystal aggregation, and epitaxy. In this scheme,[21,22] renal stones
form by *nucleation* of the crystal nidus from a supersaturated solution, followed by growth of the nidus into stone through processes
of *crystal growth*, *epitaxial growth*, and *crystal aggregation*. This
scheme is consistent with either the precipitation–crystallization
theory or the matrix theory, since the same principles apply
whether stones form without or within organic matrix. The relevance of the inhibitor theory is obvious, since inhibitors may be
present for each step of stone formation, from crystal nidation to
growth of nidus. It is recognized that promoters of these processes
may be present in urine as well. The following sections will
discuss the current knowledge regarding the regulation of these
processes in detail.

PROCESS OF NUCLEATION

Nucleation describes the process by which crystal nidus is
formed.[21,23] It may be defined by the measure of the urinary state
of saturation and of the limit of metastability with respect to the
crystal nidus. The nidus forms when the sample is oversaturated,[24]
i.e., when the extent of supersaturation exceeds the metastable
limit.

State of Saturation

It is generally recognized that urinary activity products[1,2] of constituent ions of stones potentially provide the best estimates of the state of saturation. The concentration product, or the concentration of individual ions such as Ca or oxalate, generally gives a poor measure of urinary saturation. The ionic activity is a function not only of total concentration, but also of pH-dependent dissociation, ion-pair formation,[1] and ionic strength.

Relative Saturation Ratio. Although several techniques for estimating the state of saturation have been reported, they differ in methodology and have yielded varying results. Three general approaches have been introduced. In one approach, utilized by Robertson et al.[1] and Finlayson et al.,[25] the activity product is calculated from a careful estimation of ionic activities in urine and compared with the thermodynamic solubility product obtained in simple aqueous solutions. The ratio of the activity product (A_i) and the thermodynamic solubility product (A_o) yielded the relative solution ratio.[26] This approach may be illustrated by the method of Robertson et al.[1] for calculating the relative saturation ratio for Ca oxalate. The ionic strength and the extent of dissociation of oxalate were estimated from direct analysis of concentrations of calcium, magnesium, sodium, potassium, ammonium, phosphate, oxalate, sulfate, and citrate, and from pH and known dissociation constants. The amounts of soluble complexes formed among these constituents were calculated from the stability constants; these complexes included $CaHPO_4$, $MgHPO_4$, $NaHPO_4^-$, $KHPO_4^-$, $CaH_2PO_4^+$, HOx^-, $CaOx$, $MgOx$, $HCitrate^{2-}$, $H_2Citrate^-$, $CaCitrate^-$, $MgHCitrate$, $MgCitrate^-$, $NaCitrate^{2-}$, $CaSO_4$, $MgSO_4$, $NaSO_4^-$, and KSO_4^-. The "ionic" concentrations of Ca and oxalate were determined by subtracting the amounts of soluble complexes from total concentrations. The product of molar ionic concentration and the respective activity coefficients, obtained from the ionic strength from the modification of the Debye-Hückel equation, yielded the ionic activities. To obtain thermodynamic solubility products of Ca oxalate, synthetic Ca oxalate was incubated to equilibrium in an artificial solution of known ionic composition, and the activity product of Ca^{2+} and $(COO)_2{}^{2-}$ was obtained.

A major problem with this technique is that A_i is obtained in complex solutions (urine), whereas A_o is determined in simple solutions.[26] Because of the inherent complexity of urine, errors may be introduced during estimation in urine of ionic strength and of ionic concentrations of Ca^{2+} and $(COO)_2{}^{2-}$. In contrast to situations in simple solutions, there may be other chelators of Ca and oxalate in urine, which this calculation may not recognize. The failure to account for these soluble complexes will give higher than actual concentrations of these ionic constituents. Thus, although the thermodynamic solubility product (A_o) may be accurately determined, the activity product (A_i) may be overestimated. This finding is probably the basis for the recent demonstration that A_i/A_o may overestimate the state of saturation of Ca oxalate in urine.[26]

Activity Product Ratio. In another approach, the activity product ratio (APR), utilized by Pak[2] and Pak and Holt,[3] the solubility of the solid phase was determined experimentally in each urine sample. Thus, the activity products were calculated for the same urine samples before and after incubation of urine to steady state with a synthetic solid phase, against which the state of saturation was being measured, to yield A_i and A_o', respectively. The initial activity product (A_i) was then compared with A_o', rather than A_o. The state of saturation was represented by A_i/A_o', or APR, a value of 1 indicating saturation, a value of greater than 1 supersaturation, and a value of less than 1 undersaturation.

Advantages of the approach utilizing the APR are as follows[26]: First, it may eliminate certain errors inherent in the calculation of relative saturation ratio, e.g., in the calculation of soluble complexes and of ionic strength. Since identical methods are used in calculating activity products in initial and final urine, the same errors may contribute to the derivation of A_i as contribute to the derivation of A_o'. These errors, including those resulting from complex formation, may be "canceled" when the activity products are taken as the ratio (A_i/A_o').

Second, it provides a "direct" assessment of supersaturation or undersaturation from the extent to which the synthetic solid phase undergoes growth or dissolution in urine. The APR has a physicochemical "reality," because it indicates the extent to which the synthetic solid phase undergoes growth or dissolution in urine.[2] Thus, when a urine sample was supersaturated (APR > 1), there was growth of the solid phase, as indicated by decreases in concentrations of constituent ions in the ambient fluid. Conversely, when a urine sample was undersaturated (APR < 1), there was a dissolution of the solid phase, since the concentration of constituent ions in the ambient fluid increased.

The following requirements must be satisfied for the method to be valid[26]: First, it is necessary to show experimentally that the fraction of soluble complexes involving ionic constituents of stones is not significantly changed following incubation. In the studies with brushite,[26] the fraction of bound Ca or of bound HPO_4 did not change following incubation. Moreover, in urine samples containing less than 5 mM Ca and 0.5 mM oxalate, the fraction of bound Ca or of bound oxalate did not change significantly following incubation with Ca oxalate.[26] The bound fraction therefore canceled out during the calculation of the APR (A_i/A_o').

Second, the solid phase must be completely separated from ambient solution following incubation in urine. The need was met by passage through a Millipore filter (0.05 μm). Finally, an equilibrium between the solid phase and urine must be reached. Because of crystal growth inhibitors in urine, the attainment of equilibrium may be considerably delayed. Moreover, if an insufficient amount of the solid phase is added, the crystals may be covered by a film of inhibitors and may attain a new "equilibrium" state. These effects of inhibitors may be overcome by using an excess of the solid phase.[3] For example, A_o' was considerably higher than A_o when it was measured in a supersaturated synthetic medium containing diphosphonate (2 mg P/liter) following addition of a small amount of Ca oxalate (0.5 mg/liter).[8] However, when the same medium containing diphosphonate was incubated with the larger amount of Ca oxalate (10 mg/ml), A_o' approximated A_o.

Despite these precautions, the inhibitor activity may not be totally removed and the true equilibrium state may never be reached in complex solutions such as urine. Since inhibitors of both crystal growth and crystal dissolution may be present, the experimentally derived solubility product (A_o') may be greater than the true solubility product at equilibrium in supersaturated samples, equal to the true product in saturated solutions, and less than the true product in undersaturated samples. Thus, the failure to reach true equilibrium during incubation with the solid phase may result in an APR that underestimates the extent of supersaturation and overestimates the degree of undersaturation. However, the APR should indicate saturation in saturated solutions. It is clear, therefore, that the technique utilizing the APR will provide a qualitatively valid assessment of the state of saturation, even when true equilibrium is not reached.

Comparison of Relative Saturation Ratio and Activity Product Ratio (Table II). The APR is independent of the particular method utilized for the calculation of activity product. Thus, essentially the same values for the APR of Ca oxalate in urine were obtained whether the methods of Robertson *et al.*,[1] Finlayson *et al.*,[25] or Pak and Holt[3] were utilized (Figure 2).[26] In contrast, these

TABLE II. Comparison of Relative Saturation Ratio and Activity Product Ratio

	Relative saturation ratio	Activity product ratio
Initial activity product (A_i) is compared with . . .	. . . thermodynamic solubility product (A_o)	. . . experimentally derived solubility in urine (A_o')
Soluble complexes . . .	. . . need to be accurately determined	. . . may be "canceled"
May overestimate the extent of . . .	. . . supersaturation, undersaturation, saturation	. . . undersaturation
May underestimate the extent of . . .	—	. . . supersaturation
Correctly estimates . . .	—	. . . saturation
Accuracy depends on . . .	. . . analysis of all soluble complexes	. . . incubation of solid phase to "equilibrium," and complete removal of solid phase following incubation

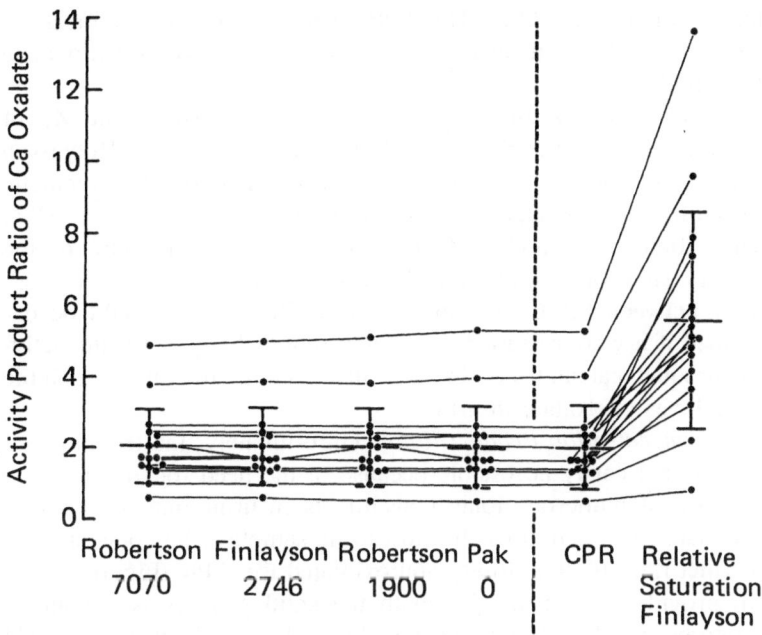

FIGURE 2. Comparison of activity product ratios of Ca oxalate obtained with four methods—Robertson (7070), Finlayson (2746), Robertson (1900), and Pak (0)—with concentration product ratio (CPR) and relative saturation ratio. Lines connecting points indicate studies on the same urine sample. The relative saturation ratio is the ratio of the initial activity product of Ca oxalate obtained by Finlayson (2746) and the K_{sp}. Horizontal bars indicate means $\pm$ 1 S.D. of 16 samples.

methods yielded widely differing relative saturation ratios.[26] The relative saturation ratio (A_i/A_o) of Ca oxalate obtained in the same samples was higher than the APR (A_i/A_o'). From the foregoing discussion, it may be concluded that the relative saturation ratio probably overestimates the state of saturation with respect to Ca oxalate. This conclusion is supported by the observation that in some urine samples that were estimated to be supersaturated by the technique of relative saturation ratio, a dissolution of the added solid phase occurred, as reflected by undersaturation according to calculation utilizing the APR. The APR currently provides the most accurate and reliable measure of the state of saturation of Ca oxalate in urine.[26]

Unlike the results for the Ca oxalate system, the A_o' of brushite obtained in urine (according to the technique of Robertson *et al.*[1]) did not differ significantly from the A_o derived in synthetic medium, and the relative saturation ratio approximated the APR. Thus, both A_i/A_o and A_i/A_o' provided a reliable measure of the urinary state of saturation with respect to brushite. The discrepancy between the Ca oxalate and brushite systems could be explained if it were assumed that the current techniques for the activity product calculations do not fully account for all the soluble complexes of oxalate in urine.

Concentration Product Ratio. Unfortunately, the technique of APR is not easily accessible because of the need for the chemical analysis of numerous ionic constituents in urine and the need to calculate ionic activities. In most urine samples, the concentration product ratio (CPR) closely approximated the APR (Figures 2 and 3), provided the incubation with the solid phase was conducted properly and the pH was kept within 0.1 unit of the original pH during incubation.[26,27] This approach is simple, since it does not require the calculation of activity products. For example, the determination of the CPR of Ca oxalate requires only the analysis of total Ca and total oxalate before and following incubation with Ca oxalate. The ratio of molar concentration product of Ca and oxalate in the original sample and the corresponding value in the urine filtrate following incubation yields the CPR. Unless a very high accuracy is desired, the CPR may be used to estimate the state of saturation with respect to brushite, Ca oxalate, and monosodium urate in most urine samples (Ca <5 mM, oxalate <0.5 mM).

Clinical Relevance of the State of Saturation. The approach utilizing the APR segregated ''non-stone-forming'' urine from ''stone-forming'' urine.[3] Urine samples from control subjects were found to be invariably undersaturated with respect to brushite, whereas samples from patients with hypercalciuria and Ca urolithiasis were usually supersaturated[2,3,7,28] (Figure 4). Among control subjects, urine samples were undersaturated or only slightly super-

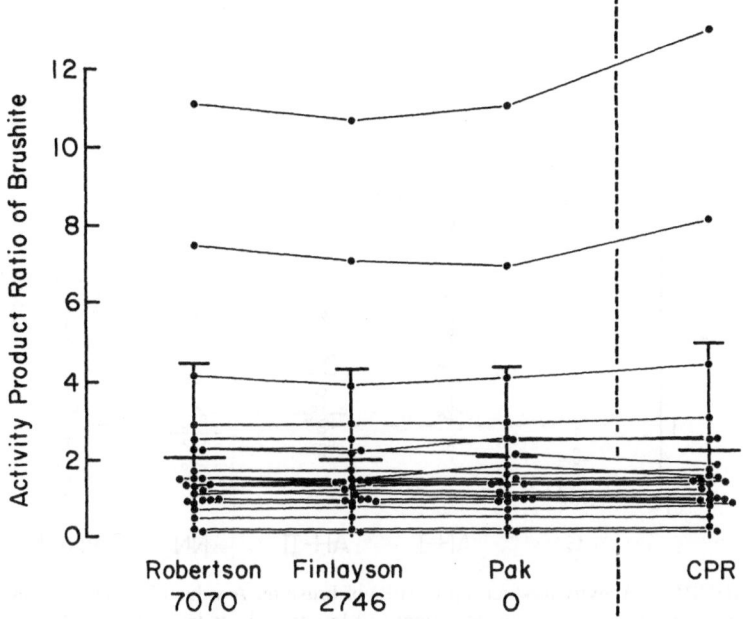

FIGURE 3. Activity product ratio and concentration product ratio (CPR) of brushite. Lines connecting points indicate studies on the same urine sample. The activity product ratio was obtained as the ratio of the activity product of the original sample and that after incubation with synthetic brushite. Horizontal bars indicate means ± 1 S.D.

saturated with respect to Ca oxalate; samples from stone-formers were almost always supersaturated (Figure 5).[3] Moreover, urine samples from patients with hyperuricosuric Ca urolithiasis were usually supersaturated with respect to monosodium urate, whereas samples from subjects with normouricosuria were undersaturated[29] [see Figure 18 (Chapter 5)].

The findings presented above clearly indicate that an initial requirement of stone formation—supersaturation with respect to stone salts—is satisfied in patients with Ca urolithiasis. It should be noted that the approach utilizing the relative saturation ratio

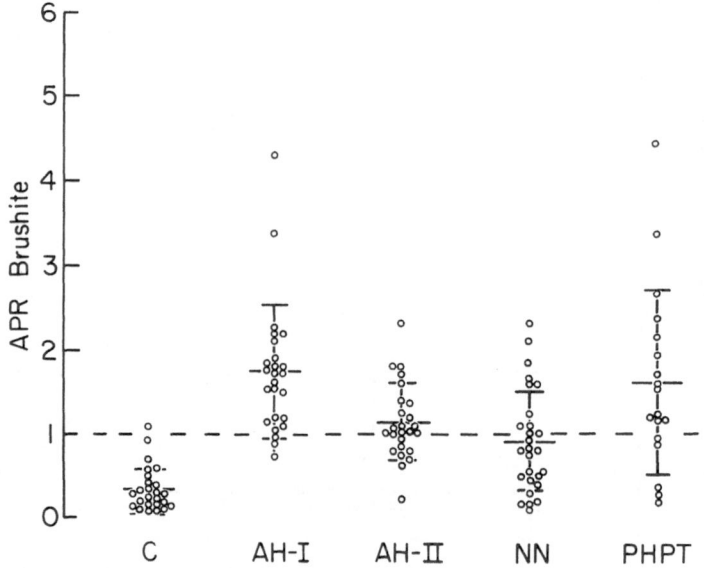

FIGURE 4. Activity product ratio (APR) of brushite. A value of 1 indicates saturation; greater than 1, supersaturation; and less than 1, undersaturation. (C) Control group; (AH-I) absorptive hypercalciuria Type I; (AH-II) absorptive hypercalciuria Type II; (NN) normocalciuric nephrolithiasis; (PHPT) primary hyperparathyroidism. Horizontal bars indicate means $\pm$ 1 S.D.

does not provide the same discrimination between stone-formers and control subjects as does the APR.[1] For example, using the relative saturation ratio, urine samples from control subjects as well as samples from stone-formers were considerably supersaturated with respect to Ca oxalate.[1,30]

Limit of Metastability

Urine supports a certain degree of metastably supersaturated state with respect to stone-forming salts.[21] Metastability may be defined as the condition in which spontaneous nucleation or precipitation of stone-forming salt does not occur, even though urine

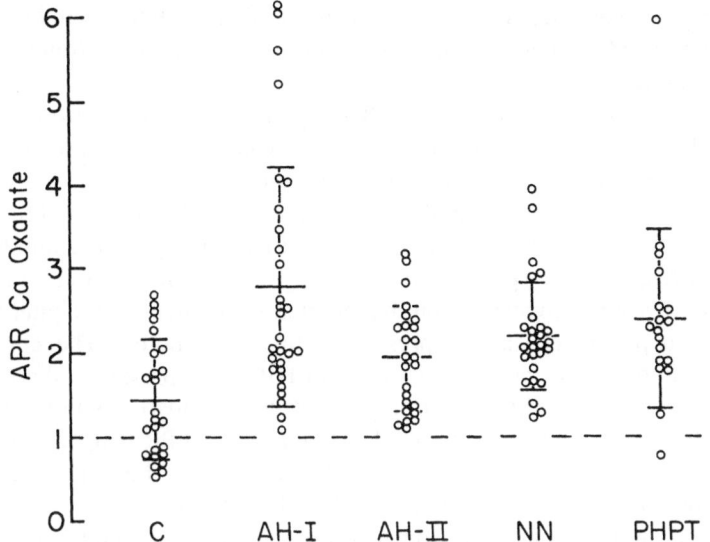

FIGURE 5. Activity product ratio (APR) of Ca oxalate. A value of 1 indicates saturation; greater than 1, supersaturation; and less than 1, undersaturation. (C) Control group; (AH-I) absorptive hypercalciuria Type I; (AH-II) absorptive hypercalciuria Type II; (NN) normocalciuric nephrolithiasis; (PHPT) primary hyperparathyroidism. Horizontal bars indicate means ± 1 S.D.

may be supersaturated with respect to that substance. This state may be illustrated by the high school chemistry experiment concerned with the solubility of sucrose. When no more sugar will dissolve in solution at room temperature, additional sugar will go into solution when the solution is heated. The sugar will remain in solution when the solution is cooled to room temperature. The solution is then metastably supersaturated with respect to sugar. However, once a scratch is made on the side of the breaker containing the sugar solution or seed crystals of sucrose are added, the excess sugar will crystallize out of solution.

The extent of metastability with respect to stone-forming salts is believed to be dependent on the inhibitors that increase it and on the promoters that reduce it. The limit of metastability indicates the point of nucleation, and may be defined by the formation product ratio.

Formation Product Ratio. The formation product ratio (FPR) is the lowest supersaturated state at which nucleation is initiated.[31-33] Above this value, nucleation proceeds. The ratio was determined as follows: For the determination of the FPR of brushite,[32] the urine sample was rendered increasingly supersaturated with respect to Ca phosphate by adding a solution of Ca chloride. The lowest Ca concentration that elicited spontaneous precipitation (of Ca phosphate) at the prescribed time was noted. The corresponding activity product of Ca^{2+} and HPO_4^{2-} represented the formation product. The formation product was compared with the activity product at saturation (A_o'). Thus, the FPR was a direct measure of the number of times the urine must be saturated to allow spontaneous precipitation. The FPR of Ca oxalate[3] was obtained similarly, after adding to urine increasing amounts of oxalate as oxalic acid or sodium oxalate. The point of nucleation in both the brushite and the Ca oxalate system was indicated by the appearance of a visible precipitate or a decline in the filtrate concentration of Ca and phosphate or oxalate. When urinary pH was less than 6.9, the precipitate formed following addition of Ca is brushite; thus, this study measures the FPR of brushite.[32]

Nature of the Nucleation Process. There is some debate as to whether the nucleation of Ca phosphate or Ca oxalate occurring in urine that is devoid of solid phase proceeds by homogeneous nucleation or by other means such as heterogeneous nucleation.[21,23] In homogeneous nucleation, crystal nuclei are formed *de novo* from constituent ions in solution without the influence of solids other than the precipitating phase. In heterogeneous nucleation, various impurities provide a foreign surface for nucleation and catalyze the reaction. Thus, the formation product or metastable limit is higher in homogeneous nucleation than in heterogeneous nucleation. Moreover, the final number of crystal particles produced may differentiate the two forms of nucleation.[23] Whereas homogeneous nucleation involves generation of new particles, heterogeneous nucleation does not create new particles, since growth occurs over foreign surfaces. The final crystal count from homogeneous nucleation is believed to be greater than 10^6 particles/ml. A particle count lower than this number probably indicates catalyzed, nonhomogeneous nucleation.[34]

Robertson[35] found that the formation product of Ca salts obtained in synthetic solutions by spontaneous precipitation at an early time period ($\leq$ 15 min) was not influenced by the presence of known inhibitors. The value representing the highest experimentally obtainable by their technique was considered to represent homogeneous nucleation. This conclusion is probably invalid for the following reasons: First, our experiments clearly indicate that the FPR of brushite or Ca oxalate or both is dependent on the presence in urine of inhibitors or promoters of nucleation, at all time periods from induction. Thus, the addition of diphosphonate (EHDP) significantly increased the FPRs within the first hour as well as after 3 days of induction.[8] The presence of a calcifiable matrix (Achilles tendon collagen) decreased the FPR of brushite, though not of Ca oxalate (Figure 6).[22] Second, the crystal particle count in urine has been reported[36] to be approximately 10^4/ml, a number too low for homogeneous nucleation. Finally, urine is probably very rich in impurities that are capable of catalyzing nucleation.[37] From these considerations, the nucleation that proceeds in urine, and that is estimated by the FPR, is probably nonhomogeneous.

Clinical Relevance of the Formation Product Ratio. The FPRs are generally obtained after 3 hr of induction from urine filtrate in the absence of solid phase at 37°C.[3] The absolute value of this ratio may not be biologically relevant, since the 3 hr of induction probably does not correspond to the time required for nucleation to take place in the urinary tract *in vivo,* and the participation of the calcifiable organic matrix may have been excluded. Moreover, the FPR is usually measured in urine samples obtained under optimal conditions of high fluid intake and low Ca intake. The value of the FPR derives from its usefulness in comparing the extent of inhibition or promotion of nucleation in stone-formers and control subjects, and in assessing response to treatment. Since the FPR is dependent on inhibitor or promoter activity, it must be

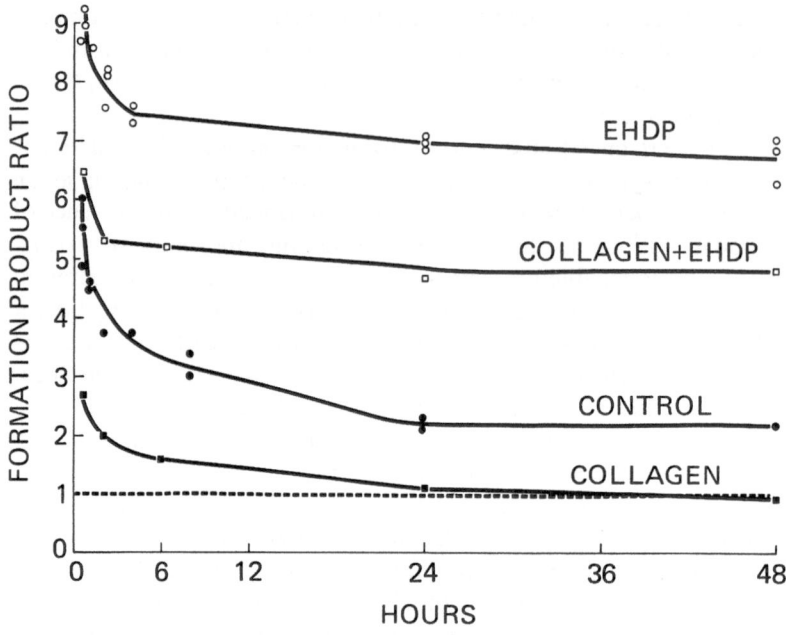

FIGURE 6. Effect of diphosphonate (EHDP) and collagen on the formation product ratio of brushite.

measured in individual urine specimens.[3] The formation product obtained in synthetic medium[1] probably has limited clinical relevance.

In most control urine samples and in many samples from stone-formers, the FPRs of brushite and Ca oxalate were higher than the corresponding values obtained in a simple synthetic medium in the absence of inhibitors or promoters [see Figure 16 (Chapter 4)].[3] The results indicated the presence in urine of inhibitors of nucleation. However, in some control urine samples, and in many samples from stone-formers, the FPRs of brushite and Ca oxalate were less than the corresponding values obtained in synthetic medium.[3] The results cannot be accounted for entirely by the absence or deficiency of inhibitors of nucleation. The inhibitor typically increases the FPRs of brushite and Ca oxalate. If the inhibitor activity were the sole factor controlling the FPR, the values of the FPR in urine would have approached those in synthetic solutions, but would not have fallen below them in the absence or lack of inhibitors. The results indicate that the nucleation of brushite and Ca oxalate may have been promoted in certain specimens, particularly from stone-formers. The nature of the soluble "promoter" is not known. The promoter activity supports the probable participation in nonhomogeneous nucleation of noncrystalline components in urine, as will be discussed. These studies do not exclude the concurrent role of absence or deficiency of inhibitors of nucleation.

Estimation of Propensity for Nucleation. The formulation of techniques for the APR and FPR has allowed a quantitative assessment of the propensity for the nucleation of brushite and Ca oxalate. In this schematic diagram (Figure 7),[22] the state of saturation

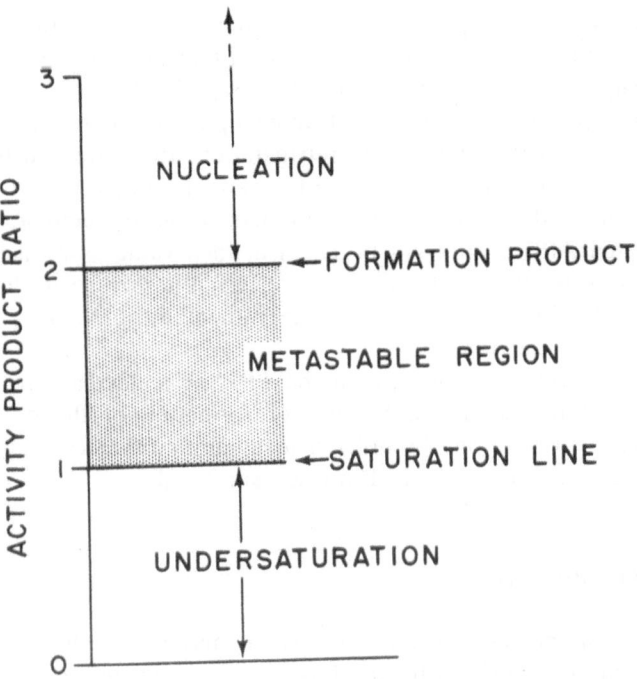

FIGURE 7. Schematic diagram for the formation of the crystal nidus.

with respect to the solid phase is indicated by the APR. An APR of 1 indicates saturation. Points below this line represent undersaturation; those above, supersaturation. The shaded area between saturation and twice saturation indicates a metastably supersaturated state. In this region, even though urine specimens may be as much as twice saturated with respect to the solid phase, nucleation does not take place. The point at which nucleation commences is the FPR. Above the FPR, nucleation takes place. This is the area of oversaturation.

The value of this scheme lies in its usefulness in predicting the likelihood of nucleation, and in quantitating response to treatment. A reduction in the FPR, as by the presence of promoter or a deficiency of inhibitors, or an increase in the APR (state of saturation), will increase the likelihood of formation of the crystal nidus. According to this scheme, stone-forming urine samples have a greater propensity for stone formation because they are usually supersaturated[2,3] and possess a lower limit of metastability,[3] as shown previously. (It should be recognized that in actual practice, the urinary saturation seldom exceeds the limit of metastability. The urine specimens are collected under optimal conditions, particularly of high fluid intake and refrigeration, to assure that they are not oversaturated. In fact, the FPR cannot be determined experimentally if the sample is oversaturated. Thus, the comparison of FPR and APR should not be taken at face value as an actual reflection of the physicochemical state of urine in the urinary tract; rather, it should be regarded as a measure of the propensity for spontaneous nucleation.)

Alternatively, an increase in the FPR or a decrease in the APR should reduce the probability of formation of the crystal nidus. This scheme may be utilized to quantitate the response to treatment, as will be illustrated in Chapters 3 and 4.

CRYSTAL GROWTH

Once the crystal nidus has formed, it may grow into a stone of the same composition by the process of crystal growth if the urine is supersaturated with respect to the crystal nidus. Crystal growth may be measured by adding to urine a small amount of synthetic solid phase (representing stone) and by determining the rate of its growth.[3-5,38,39] Since crystal growth is influenced by the amount of solid phase added, the duration of growth, and the extent of metastable supersaturation, these variables must be controlled. Crystal growth may be determined from the decreases in filtrate concentrations of constituent ions of stone for which growth is being measured.

Assessment of Crystal Growth in Whole Urine. Techniques for the quantitative assessment of the crystal growth of brushite and Ca oxalate, applicable to undiluted whole urine, have been devised.[3] For measurement of the crystal growth of Ca oxalate, a small amount of the solid phase of Ca oxalate monohydrate (0.5 mg/ml) was added to several solutions with varying degrees of metastable supersaturation (the solutions having been rendered supersaturated by addition of a solution of sodium oxalate). After 30 min of incubation, the crystal growth was measured from the decrease in the total concentration of Ca and oxalate in the filtrate. There was a linear relationship between crystal growth and the extent of supersaturation, with zero growth at saturation. Thus, only one value for crystal growth needs to be determined for each urine sample, since values at any state of saturation may be estimated by interpolation. The interpolated value at sixfold saturation (APR of 6) was calculated in urine samples. Thus, crystal growth of Ca oxalate represented the amount of Ca and oxalate deposited over 0.5 mg/ml of the seed of Ca oxalate monohydrate over 30 min from urine samples sixfold saturated with respect to Ca oxalate.

The crystal growth of brushite was calculated by a similar technique from the fall in the concentration of Ca and phosphate at 30 min.[3] A greater amount of brushite (2.5 mg/ml) was required because of larger crystallite size. The interpolated value at threefold saturation was utilized.

This method, applicable to whole urine, requires the use of relatively large amounts of the solid phase. When smaller amounts are used, the crystal growth is often too slow to be accurately measured. Unfortunately, the use of larger amounts of seed distorts the kinetics of growth, and may not provide full inhibitor activity, since certain inhibitors may be absorbed on the seed crystals. For the Ca oxalate system, for example, the reaction is probably first-order,[3] rather than second-order, as has been reported.[4,5,38]

Crystal Growth in Diluted Urine. When smaller amounts of seed (e.g., <0.1 mg/ml) are used in synthetic medium, the crystal growth of Ca oxalate is found to be second-order,[4,5,38] whereas that of brushite is first-order.[39]

The method described above has been modified to assess growth of Ca oxalate in urine.[4,5] It consists of measurement of crystal growth at various dilutions of urine in known synthetic medium. The crystal growth of Ca oxalate may be described by the rate law

$$dC/dt = k(C - C_\infty)^2$$

where C and C_∞ are free ionic activities of calcium at time t and at saturation, respectively. The rate constant k for each diluted sample may be derived from the integrated form of the above equation, whereby a plot of t vs. $1/(C - C_\infty)$ yields a straight line of slope k. The degree of dilution required to reduce crystal growth by 50%, which may be obtained by interpolation, gave a measure of crystal growth.[5] Employing this technique, Meyer and Smith[5] found a potent inhibitor activity in urine; a urine sample diluted 62-fold gave a 50% inhibition of Ca oxalate crystal growth.

This technique is clearly superior to the technique described for whole urine in the assessment of inhibitor activity of isolated urinary components. Because of potent urinary inhibitor activity, however, it probably provides a reflection of inhibitor activity in diluted urine, not in whole urine.

Clinical Relevance of Crystal Growth. Our technique,[3] though probably less valid by kinetic and physicochemical criteria than that of Meyer and Smith,[5] provides a measure of inhibitor (or promoter) activity in whole urine. Using this procedure, we found the crystal growth of brushite and Ca oxalate to be significantly elevated in the urine of certain stone-forming groups, particularly those with primary hyperparathyroidism.[3] It is not known whether this increase is the consequence of deficiency of inhibitor or presence of promoters.

CRYSTAL AGGREGATION

Crystal aggregation describes the process by which preformed crystals aggregate into large clusters. Unlike the case with crystal growth, there is no increase in crystal mass. Crystal aggregates of Ca oxalate 100–200 μm wide have been found in stone-forming urine.[36,40] It has been postulated that normal urine contains certain substances that inhibit the aggregation of Ca oxalate crystals, thereby allowing ready passage through the urinary tract even when crystals form. Such inhibitor activity was believed to be deficient in stone-forming urine. There is some evidence that acid mucopolysaccharide may account for this inhibitor activity.[40] EHDP, which inhibits nucleation and crystal growth, has also been shown to retard crystal aggregation.[41]

Unfortunately, the methods for assessing crystal aggregation in urine have been deficient. Crystal aggregation has been measured by size distribution (in a Coulter counter),[36] or from the rate of filtration of crystal suspension through a filter of limited pore size under constant pressure (in an agglometer).[42] A typical method for the crystal aggregation of Ca oxalate employed a standard synthetic solution metastably supersaturated with respect to Ca oxalate, to which seed crystals were added and allowed to grow and aggregate. The activity in urine was determined from the changes in crystal size distribution[36] after addition of urine (1–3% by volume) to the synthetic medium. Herein lies the problem. The system represented processes of both crystal growth and aggregation. Moreover, the study employed a markedly diluted urine, a situation that may have no biological relevance. This potentially important process should be reexamined utilizing unaltered urine with pure crystal aggregation systems.

Studies utilizing the saturation–inhibition index suffer from the same limitation as the studies of crystal aggregation.[43] This index, which is a function of inhibitory activity of crystal aggregation and urinary saturation, expresses the risk of forming large crystals. While it discriminates stone-forming urine from non-stone-forming urine very well, it may have limited biological significance, since the inhibitory activity was obtained with diluted urine (1% vol/vol) and the activity product used probably overestimated the degree of saturation.[26]

HETEROGENEOUS NUCLEATION

The role of noncrystalline impurities in initiating heterogeneous nucleation of Ca salts in urine will be discussed later. This section discusses the role of heterologous crystal nuclei. In heterogeneous nucleation, nucleation from a metastably supersaturated solution is induced by a heterologous "seed." This process may underlie the mechanism for the formation of stones of mixed crystalline composition. Since the solution is metastable, the spontaneous precipitation would not have occurred during the specified period without seeding, despite supersaturation. There should be some degree of specificity to the heterogeneous nucleation for it to be biologically meaningful. Heterogeneous nucleation may occur "nonspecifically," e.g., Ca oxalate depositing over cotton fiber, provided the amount of the seed is large and the extent of metastability is high.

Several "meaningful" forms of heterogeneous nucleation, involving crystal constituents of stones, have been described.[44-47] For many systems, epitaxial fit or crystalline spatial conformity between the seed crystal and the induced phase had been demonstrated.[48] The simplest method used relies on measurement of the changes in filtrate concentration of constituent ions of the induced phase following seeding of metastably supersaturated solution (with respect to the induced phase) with a heterologous nidus.

Role of Brushite Nidus. There is some evidence suggesting that brushite ($CaHPO_4 \cdot 2H_2O$) may be the initial crystal nidus for certain Ca-containing renal stones. The potential importance of brushite was indicated by several morphological studies of both

large and small stones. The central core of large stones has sometimes been identified as Ca phosphate.[15,49] Among small stones
(<2 mm in diameter), including those composed principally of Ca
oxalate, the nidus of Ca phosphate of less than 40 μm in diameter
has been identified by electron-probe analysis.[50] The identification
of apatite as the predominant Ca phosphate phase in stones does
not necessarily exclude an important role for brushite, since
brushite may have formed first and been later transformed to hydroxyapatite.[32]

Brushite is in fact the stable phase of Ca phosphate in the normal acid pH of urine (pH <6.9). At pH greater than 6.9, brushite
undergoes a rapid transformation into Ca phosphates of higher
Ca/P ratio, such as hydroxyapatite.[32] Brushite has previously been
shown to be the predominant solid phase formed from urine under
the influence of an organic matrix[51] or by spontaneous precipitation,[32] a finding that is compatible with either the precipitation–crystallization or the matrix theory. The calcification of the
model organic matrix (Achilles tendon collagen) occurred in urine
specimens that were supersaturated with respect to brushite, but
not in an undersaturated sample.[51] The molar Ca/P ratio of the
solid phase of the "calcified" matrix approximated the theoretical
value of 1 for brushite, and was identified as brushite by X-ray
diffraction. The precipitates, obtained spontaneously on addition
of Ca chloride in urine samples with a pH less than 6.9, were identified as brushite; at pH greater than 6.9, they were apatite.[32]

It has been argued that brushite cannot serve as a nidus for
stones because of the infrequent occurrence of brushite stones.[52]
This fact probably reflects the hydrolysis of brushite to compounds
of higher Ca/P ratio, which occurs rapidly in an alkaline pH. The
preponderance of renal stones of higher Ca/P ratio such as apatite
is not surprising, because the passage of alkaline urine during the
course of the stone disease is not uncommon.

The brushite nidus may account for the formation of apatite
and certain Ca oxalate stones. Apatite stones may form from alkaline transformation of brushite. Even at persistently alkaline pH,
the possibility that brushite is formed before hydroxyapatite cannot

be excluded. There is some evidence that brushite may represent the logical precursor in the formation of hydroxyapatite at alkaline pH.[53]

Several forms of heterogeneous nucleation have been implicated in the formation of Ca oxalate stones from brushite nidus. First, brushite seed may induce crystallization of Ca oxalate.[7] Second, brushite may be transformed to hydroxyapatite first; hydroxyapatite may then cause heterogeneous nucleation of Ca oxalate.[46] (Indeed, there is some evidence that hydroxyapatite is more efficient than brushite in inducing heterogeneous nucleation of Ca oxalate.) Finally, brushite may induce nucleation of monosodium urate.[46] The urate salt so formed may lead to Ca oxalate crystallization.[44,45]

Two clinical studies have provided indirect support for the pathogenetic role of brushite nidus in Ca oxalate stone formation. The positive clinical response (decrease in incidence of stone episodes) to treatment with sodium cellulose phosphate is best correlated with the fall in the urinary APR of brushite, rather than of Ca oxalate.[9,11] Moreover, the FPR of brushite is considerably less than that of Ca oxalate[3]; thus, nucleation of brushite may be more likely than nucleation of Ca oxalate. Finally, the discrimination between stone-forming urine and control urine is better provided by the APR of brushite than by the APR of Ca oxalate.[1,3,30]

Role of Monosodium Urate Nidus. Recent studies suggest that seed of monosodium urate may induce heterogeneous nucleation of Ca salts.[44-46] This process has been implicated as one of the mechanisms for the formation of Ca stones in patients with hyperuricosuria,[29] as will be discussed in Chapter 5. Solid seeds of monosodium urate (as little as 0.1 mg/ml of solution) caused prompt crystallization of Ca oxalate and of Ca phosphate from solutions that were metastably supersaturated with respect to these Ca salts (Figure 8). These effects were found at both low and high pHs (5.3–7.4). On the other hand, uric acid seed was incapable of producing heterogeneous nucleation of Ca oxalate or Ca phosphate except at high pH (≥ 6.7).[46] The positive effect found for uric acid may be the result of monosodium urate that had formed from uric acid at high pH (see Chapter 5 for further discussion).

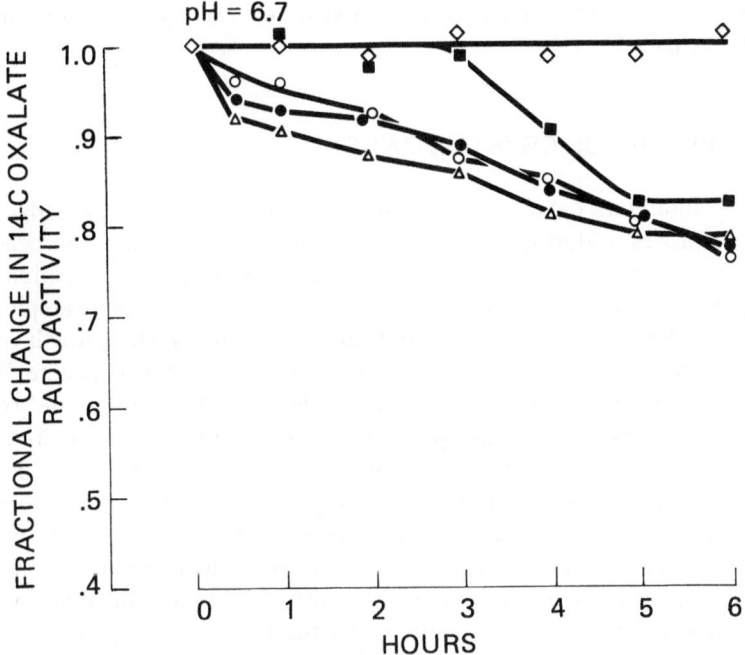

FIGURE 8. Heterogeneous nucleation of Ca oxalate by seed of monosodium urate (NaH urate). (◇) None; (■) 0.1 mg/ml; (○) 0.5 mg/ml; (●) 2 mg/ml; (△) 5 mg/ml.

Clinical Relevance of Heterogeneous Nucleation. The results cited above indicate that heterogeneous nucleation may play an important role in the formation of stones of mixed crystalline composition. This conclusion has been questioned, however, on several grounds. First, heterogeneous nucleation has usually been tested in artificial media, not in urine, and the same form or degree of heterogeneous nucleation may not proceed in urine because of inhibitor activity. The effect of various inhibitors on heterogeneous nucleation has not been systematically examined. If these inhibitors are present in urine, it is not known whether their activity is modified in stone-forming urine. Second, the rate of crystal growth by heterogeneous nucleation may be too slow to establish the nidus in the urinary tract.[34]

INHIBITORS OF CRYSTALLIZATION

Inhibitors have been identified at each step of the crystallization process—during nucleation, crystal growth, crystal aggregation, heterogeneous nucleation, and crystalline phase transition. The effect of certain inhibitors may be generalized. For example, EHDP has been shown to inhibit nucleation and crystal growth of brushite[54] and Ca oxalate,[8] crystal aggregation of Ca oxalate,[41] heterogeneous nucleation of Ca oxalate by hydroxyapatite or monosodium urate,[55] and phase transition of brushite to hydroxyapatite.[56] The effect of other inhibitors may be more specific, localized to a particular step in the crystallization process, or to a particular crystalline constituent. These inhibitors may operate either in the presence or in the absence of the organic matrix.

Historical Considerations. The role of inhibitors in stone formation received a big impetus when the concept of "good" and "evil" urine* was introduced in 1959 by Thomas and Howard.[57] It was found that the urine of stone-formers calcified the rat rachitic cartilage, whereas that of non-stone-formers did not. These workers subsequently identified a factor in urine that inhibited calcification. They found it to be composed of two peptides[19]: peptide B, which had a molecular weight of approximately 500, and peptide C, which had a molecular weight of approximately 1000. As assayed by the cartilage calcification system, peptide B was found to be about five times more potent on a weight basis than was pyrophosphate in inhibiting calcification. Peptide C was equivalent to pyrophosphate in potency.

---

*The concept of "good" and "evil" urine generated the following anecdote: The defeat of Germany during World War I was partly attributed to the passage of "good" urine by the German soldiers. Allegedly, the German soldiers, unable to get to restrooms readily because of constant shelling by the Allies, urinated on the freshly built concrete bunkers. Since their "good" urine kept the concrete from solidifying, the bunkers became easy prey to shelling by the Allies.

Unfortunately, even if these inhibitory peptides exist, it is doubtful that they play a significant role in the formation of renal stones. First, the studies of inhibition conducted by these workers may be of limited biological significance, since they were performed with altered urine specimens that were adjusted to a pH of 7.4 and diluted to a specific gravity of 1.010.[2] Second, these investigators made no attempt to correlate the calcification process with the state of saturation of urine with respect to any solid phase. Thus, their studies do not clearly exclude the possibility that the calcification of rachitic cartilage by stone-forming urine may have resulted from the urinary supersaturation, rather than from a deficiency of the inhibitors of calcification. Finally, it was shown that the total "inhibitor activity" in normal urine may be accounted for by the usual urinary constituents, not necessarily by the peptides.[58]

Even though the role of urinary peptides may have been discounted, it is generally believed that urine possesses potent inhibitor activity. Substances reported to have inhibitor action range from pyrophosphate[18] and macromolecules (including mucopolysaccharide)[40] to citrate, magnesium, and zinc.[59]

Clinical Relevance of Inhibitors. Any scheme implicating an important pathogenetic role for inhibitors in stone formation assumes that the inhibitors are deficient in amount or activity in the urine of patients with stones. Robertson *et al.*[40] have reported that the activity of inhibitor(s) of Ca oxalate aggregation is less in stone-forming urine than in control urine. In a preliminary study, Fleisch[60] has found total urinary pyrophosphate excretion to be reduced in male subjects with "idiopathic" Ca urolithiasis. However, renal excretions of many inhibitors, including citrate, magnesium, and zinc, have not been found to be reduced in stone-formers.

PROMOTERS OF CRYSTALLIZATION

Promoters are substances that facilitate the crystallization process. In a broad sense, the heterologous crystal nidus involved in heterogeneous nucleation represents a promoter. However, this

section considers the role of only soluble and insoluble noncrystalline substances. Their clinical relevance is obvious, since stone
formation may be the consequence of the presence of promoters
in urine, rather than of deficiency of inhibitors. Like inhibitors,
promoters presumably influence every step in the crystallization
process.

Research relevant to promoters is in its infancy. No authentic
natural promoter has yet been identified. Only a few probable examples of promotion of crystallization have been recognized. First,
the FPRs of brushite and Ca oxalate were significantly reduced and
crystal growth was significantly increased in urine samples from
certain stone-formers.[3] This finding suggested the presence of a
soluble promoter that facilitated nucleation and crystal growth.
Second, the addition of a model organic matrix (Achilles tendon
collagen) lowered the FPR of brushite, the result indicating promotion of nucleation (see Figure 6).[22,51] A preliminary study indicates that a certain organic matrix isolated from stones possesses
a similar promoter activity. The results suggest an important etiological role for organic matrix in stone formation.

ORGANIC MATRIX OF STONES

The role of promoters of nucleation in stone formation has
long been espoused by Boyce and co-workers[15-17] in their matrix
theory. Virtually all renal stones were shown to contain a proteinaceous organic matrix. Structural studies of renal stones suggested that the process of stone formation may require the presence
of mucoproteins. The most prominent antigenic component of the
organic matrix of stones has been identified by Boyce and associ-
ates as matrix substance A. This substance has been found in the
urine of patients with large bilateral or rapidly recurrent renal
calculi, but never in the urine of non-stone-forming subjects. Recently, intranephronic calculosis has been identified in the renal
tubules of patients with renal calculi.[61] These intranephronic bodies appear to resemble microspherules or Ca-containing bodies in
the ultrafiltrate ($< 10,000$ daltons) of stone-forming urine. The ab-

sence of intranephronic calculosis and microspherules in non-stone-forming subjects suggests a potential etiological role for these substances in stone formation. Although the chemical nature of the microspherules has not been identified, they are believed to be low-molecular-weight proteins. The proteinaceous nature of the organic matrix of stones and of microspherules raises an interesting speculation as to whether these components might have any resemblance to the γ-carboxyglutamic acid-containing proteins found in bone,[62,63] prothrombin,[64] and calcified tissues.[65] The Gla-containing proteins have been shown to possess Ca-binding capacities, and may contribute to the calcification process. Although the studies cited above suggest that the organic matrix may participate in stone formation, their ability to promote crystallization of stone-forming salts has not been directly shown.

FUTURE RESEARCH IN THE PHYSICAL CHEMISTRY OF STONE FORMATION

It has been customary to search for physicochemical factors in urine passed by the patient and to extrapolate from them the propensity for stone formation *in vivo*. Future work must consider the site of crystal formation and the ionic composition at that site.

Current techniques should be improved and new methods developed for the assessment of various steps in the crystallization process in *whole* urine. Various urine factors possessing inhibitor or promoter activity should be isolated and characterized.

REFERENCES

1. Robertson, W. G., Peacock, M., and Nordin, B. E. C. 1968. Activity products in stone-forming and non-stone-forming urine. *Clin. Sci.* **34:**579–594.
2. Pak, C. Y. C. 1969 Physicochemical basis for formation of renal stones of calcium phosphate origin: Calculation of the degree of saturation of urine with respect to brushite. *J. Clin. Invest.* **48:**1914–1922.
3. Pak, C. Y. C., and Holt, K. 1976. Nucleation and growth of brushite and calcium oxalate in urine of stone-formers. *Metabolism* **25:**665–673.

4. Meyer, J. L., and Smith, L. H. 1975. Growth of calcium oxalate crystals. I. A model for urinary stone growth. *Invest. Urol.* **13**:31–35.

5. Meyer, J. L., and Smith, L. H. 1975. Growth of calcium oxalate crystals. II. Inhibition by natural urinary crystal growth inhibitors. *Invest. Urol.* **13**:36–39.

6. Marshall, R. W., and Barry, H. 1973. Urine saturation and formation of calcium-containing renal calculi: The effects of various forms of therapy. In *Urinary Calculi: Proceedings of the International Symposium on Renal Stone Research, Madrid, 1972.* L. Cifuentes Delatte, A. Rapado, and A. Hodgkinson, Eds. Karger, Basel and New York, pp. 164–169.

7. Pak, C. Y. C. 1973. Quantitative assessment of various forms of therapy for nephrolithiasis. In *Urinary Calculi: Proceedings of the International Symposium on Renal Stone Research, Madrid, 1972.* L. Cifuentes Delatte, A. Rapado, and A. Hodgkinson, Eds. Karger, Basel and New York, pp. 177–187.

8. Pak, C. Y. C., Ohata, M., and Holt, K. 1975. Effect of diphosphonate on crystallization of calcium oxalate *in vitro. Kidney Int.* **7**:154–160.

9. Hayashi, Y., Kaplan, R. A., and Pak, C. Y. C. 1975. Effect of sodium cellulose phosphate therapy on crystallization of calcium oxalate in urine. *Metabolism* **24**:1273–1278.

10. Woelfel, A., Kaplan, R. A., and Pak, C. Y. C. 1977. Effect of hydrochlorothiazide therapy on the crystallization of calcium oxalate in urine. *Metabolism* **26**:201–205.

11. Pak, C. Y. C., Delea, C. S., and Bartter, F. C. 1974. Successful treatment of recurrent nephrolithiasis (calcium stones) with cellulose phosphate. *N. Engl. J. Med.* **290**:175–180.

12. Smith, L. H. 1976. Application of physical chemistry and metabolic factors to the management of urolithiasis. In *Urolithiasis Research.* H. Fleisch, W. G. Robertson, L. H. Smith, and W. Vahlensieck, Eds. Plenum Press, New York, pp. 199–211.

13. Vermeulen, C. W., Lyon, E. S., and Fried, F. A. 1965. On the nature of the stone-forming process. *J. Urol.* **94**:176–186.

14. Vermeulen, C. W., Lyon, E. S., and Gill, W. B. 1964. Artificial urinary concretions. *Invest. Urol.* **1**:370–386.

15. Boyce, W. H., and King, J. S., Jr. 1963. Present concepts concerning the origin of matrix and stones. *Ann. N. Y. Acad. Sci.* **104**:563–578.

16. Boyce, W. H. 1968. Organic matrix of human urinary concretions. *Am. J. Med.* **45**:673–683.

17. Boyce, W. H., and Garvey, F. K. 1956. The amount and nature of the organic matrix in urinary calculi. *J. Urol.* **76**:213–227.

18. Fleisch, H., and Bisaz, S. 1962. Isolation from urine of pyrophosphate, a calcification inhibitor. *Am. J. Physiol.* **203**:671–675.

19. Howard, J. E., Thomas, W. C., Smith, L. H., Barker, L. M., and Wadkins, C. L. 1966. A urinary peptide with extraordinary inhibitory powers against

biological "calcification" (deposition) of hydroxyapatite crystals. *Trans. Assoc. Am. Physicians* **79**:137–144.

20. Howard, J. E., and Thomas, W. C., Jr. 1968. Control of crystallization in urine. *Am. J. Med.* **45**:693–699.
21. Nancollas, G. 1976. The kinetics of crystal growth and renal stone-formation. In *Urolithiasis Research*. H. Fleisch, W. G. Robertson, L. H. Smith, and W. Vahlensieck, Eds. Plenum Press, New York, pp. 5–23.
22. Pak, C. Y. C. 1976. Disorders of stone formation. In *The Kidney*. B. M. Brenner and F. C. Rector, Jr., Eds. W. B. Saunders, Philadelphia, pp. 1326–1354.
23. Walton, A. G. 1967. Nucleation. In *The Formation and Properties of Precipitates: Chemical Analysis*. P. J. Elveng and I. M. Kolthoff, Eds. Interscience Publishing, New York, pp. 1–43.
24. Hodgkinson, A., Marshall, R. W., and Cochran, M. 1971. Diurnal variations in calcium phosphate and calcium oxalate activity products in normal and stone-forming urines. *Isr. J. Med. Sci.* **73**:1230–1234.
25. Finlayson, B., Roth, R., and DuBois, L. 1973. Calcium oxalate solubility studies. In *Urinary Calculi: Proceedings of the International Symposium on Renal Stone Research, Madrid, 1972*. L. Cifuentes Delatte, A. Rapado, and A. Hodgkinson, Eds. Karger, Basel and New York, pp. 1–7.
26. Pak, C. Y. C., Hayashi, Y., Finlayson, B., and Chu, S. 1977. Estimation of the state of saturation of brushite and calcium oxalate in urine: A comparison of three methods. *J. Lab. Clin. Med.* **89**:891–901.
27. Pak, C. Y. C., and Chu, S. 1973. A simple technique for the determination of urinary state of saturation with respect to brushite. *Invest. Urol.* **11**:211–215.
28. Pak, C. Y. C., Diller, E. C., Smith, G. W. II, and Howe, E. S. 1969. Renal stones of calcium phosphate: Physicochemical basis for their formation. *Proc. Soc. Exp. Biol. Med.* **130**:753–757.
29. Pak, C. Y. C., Waters, O., Arnold, L., Holt, K., Cox, C., and Barilla, D. 1977. Mechanism for calcium urolithiasis among patients with hyperuricosuria: Supersaturation of urine with respect to monosodium urate. *J. Clin. Invest.* **59**:426–431.
30. Oreopoulos, D. G., Wilson, D. R., Husdan, H., Pylypchuk, G., and Rapoport, A. 1976. Comparison of two methods for measuring activity products of calcium salts in urine. In *Urolithiasis Research*. H. Fleisch, W. G. Robertson, L. H. Smith, and W. Vahlensieck, Eds. Plenum Press, New York, pp. 325–328.
31. Strates, B. S., Neuman, W. F., and Levinskas, G. J. 1957. The solubility of bone mineral. II. Precipitation of near-neutral solutions of calcium and phosphate. *J. Phys. Chem.* **61**:279–282.
32. Pak, C. Y. C., Eanes, E. D., and Ruskin, B. 1971. Spontaneous precipitation of brushite: Evidence that brushite is the nidus of renal stones originating as calcium phosphate. *Proc. Natl. Acad. Sci. U.S.A.* **68**:1456–1460.

33. Hlabse, T., and Walton, A. G. 1965. The nucleation of calcium phosphate from solution. *Anal. Chim. Acta* **33**:373–377.
34. Finlayson, B. 1977. Physical chemical aspects of urolithiasis. *Kidney Int.* In press.
35. Robertson, W. G. 1973. Factors affecting the precipitation of calcium phosphate *in vitro*. *Calcif. Tissue Res.* **11**:311–322.
36. Robertson, W. G. 1969. A method for measuring calcium crystalluria. *Clin. Chim. Acta* **26**:105–110.
37. Trump, B. F., Dees, J. H., and Kim, K. M. 1972. Some aspects of kidney structure and function with comments on tissue calcification in the kidney. In *Urolithiasis: Physical Aspects*. B. Finlayson, L. Hench, and L. H. Smith, Eds. National Academy of Science, Washington, D.C., pp. 1–39.
38. Nancollas, G. H., and Gardner, G. L. 1974. Kinetics of crystal growth of calcium oxalate monohydrate. *J. Cryst. Growth* **21**:267–276.
39. Marshall, R. W., and Nancollas, G. H. 1969. The kinetics of crystal growth of dicalcium phosphate dihydrate. *J. Phys. Chem.* **73**:3838–3844.
40. Robertson, W. G., Knowles, F., and Peacock, M. 1976. Urinary acid, mucopolysaccharide inhibitors of calcium oxalate crystalization. In *Urolithiasis Research*. H. Fleisch, W. G. Robertson, L. H. Smith, and W. Vahlensieck, Eds. Plenum Press, New York, pp. 331–334.
41. Robertson, W. G., Peacock, M., Marshall, R. W., and Knowles, F. 1974. The effect of ethane-1-hydroxy-1,1-diphosphonate (EHDP) on calcium oxalate crystalluria in recurrent renal stone-formers. *Clin. Sci. Mol. Med.* **27**:13–22.
42. Fleisch, H., and Monod, A. 1973. A new technique for measuring aggregation of calcium oxalate crystals *in vitro*: Effect of urine, magnesium, pyrophosphate and diphosphonates. *Urinary Calculi: International Symposium on Renal Stone Research, Madrid, 1972*. Karger, Basel, pp. 53–56.
43. Robertson, W. G., Peacock, M., Marshall, R. W., Marshall, D. H., and Nordin, B. E. C. 1976. Saturation–inhibition index as a measure of the risk of calcium oxalate stone formation in the urinary tract. *N. Engl. J. Med.* **294**:249–252.
44. Coe, F. L, Lawton, R. L., Goldstein, R. B., and Tembe, V. 1975. Sodium urate accelerates precipitation of calcium oxalate *in vitro*. *Proc. Soc. Exp. Biol. Med.* **149**:926–929.
45. Pak, C. Y. C., and Arnold, L. H. 1975. Heterogeneous nucleation of calcium oxalate by seeds of monosodium urate. *Proc. Soc. Exp. Biol. Med.* **149**:930–932.
46. Pak, C. Y. C., Hayashi, Y., and Arnold, L. H. 1976. Heterogeneous nucleation between urate, calcium phosphate and calcium oxalate. *Proc. Soc. Exp. Biol. Med.* **153**:83–87.
47. Meyer, J., Bergert, L., and Smith, H. 1977. Epitaxy in calcium phosphate–calcium oxalate crystal growth systems. In *Proceedings of an International*

Colloquium on Renal Lithiasis. B. Finlayson and W. C. Thomas, Jr., Eds. University of Florida Press, Gainesville, pp. 66–76.

48. Lonsdale, K. 1968. Human stones: Limited studies give some details of composition, rates of growth, distribution, and possible causes. *Science* **159**:1199–1207.

40. Prien, L. 1955. Studies in urolithiasis. III. Physicochemical principles in stone formation and prevention. *J. Urol* **73**:627–652.

50. Chambers, A., Hodgkinson, A., and Hornung, G. 1972. Electron probe analysis of small urinary tract calculi. *Invest. Urol.* **9**:376–384.

51. Pak, C. Y. C., and Ruskin, B. 1970. Calcification of collagen by urine *in vitro:* Dependence on the degree of saturation of urine with respect to brushite. *J. Clin. Invest.* **49**:2353–2361.

52. Prien, E. L, and Prien, E. L, Jr. 1968. Composition and structure of urinary stone. *Am. J. Med.* **45**:654–672.

53. Francis, M. D., and Webb, N. C. 1971. Hydroxyapatite formation from a hydrated calcium monohydrogen phosphate precursor. *Calcif. Tissue Res.* **6**:335–342.

54. Ohata, M., and Pak, C. Y. C. 1973. The effect of diphosphonate on calcium phosphate crystallization in urine *in vitro. Kidney Intl.* **4**:401–406.

55. Pak, C. Y. C. 1977. Physicochemical and clinical aspects of nephrolithiasis *Proceedings of an International Colloquium on Renal Lithiasis.* B. Finlayson and W. C. Thomas, Jr., Eds. University of Florida Press, Gainesville, pp. 257–275.

56. Francis, M. D., Russell, R. G. G., and Fleisch, H. 1969. Diphosphonates inhibit stone formation of calcium phosphate crystals *in vitro* and pathological calcification *in vivo. Science* **165**:1264–1266.

57. Thomas, W. C., Jr., and Howard, J. E. 1959. Studies on the mineralizing propensity of urine from patients with and without renal calculi. *Trans. Assoc. Am. Physicians* **72**:181–187.

58. Barker, L. M., Pallante, S. L., Eisenberg, H., Joule, J. A., Becker, G. L., and Howard, J. E. 1974. Simple synthetic and natural urines have equivalent anticalcifying properties. *Invest. Urol.* **12**:79–81.

59. Byrd, E. D., and Thomas, W. C., Jr. 1963. Effect of various metals on mineralization *in vitro. Proc. Soc. Exp. Biol. Med.* **112**:640–643.

60. Fleisch, H. 1977. Personal communication.

61. Boyce, W. H., Willard, J., and Prater, T. F. 1973. Intranephronic calculosis in surgical biopsies of human kidney. In *Urinary Calculi: Proceedings of the International Symposium on Renal Stone Research, Madrid, 1972.* L. Cifuentes Delatte, A. Rapado, and A. Hodgkinson, Eds. S. Karger, Basel and New York, pp. 339–346.

62. Hauschka, P. V., Lian, J. B., and Gallop, P. M. 1975. Direct identification of the calcium binding amino acid, γ-carboxyglutamic acid, in mineralized tissue. *Proc. Natl. Acad. Sci. U.S.A.* **72**:3925–3929.

63. Price, P. A., Otsuka, A. S., Poser, J. W., Kriskaponis, J., and Raman, N. 1976. Characterization of a γ-carboxyglutamic acid-containing protein from bone. *Proc. Natl. Acad. Sci. U.S.A.* **73**:1447–1451.

64. Esmon, C. T., Sadowski, J. A., and Suttie, J. W. 1975. A new carboxylation reaction: The vitamin K-dependent incorporation of $H^{14}CO_2$ into prothrombin. *J. Biol. Chem.* **250**:4744–4748.

65. Lian, J. B., Skinner, M., Glimcher, M. J., and Gallop, P. 1976. The presence of γ-carboxyglutamic acid in the proteins associated with ectopic calcification. *Biochem. Biophys. Res. Commun.* **73**:349–355.

Chapter 3

Hypercalciurias

Hypercalciuria is probably the most common biochemical abnormality in patients with Ca urolithiasis.[1-3] Although reported estimates vary, hypercalciuria may be found in the majority of patients suffering from Ca stones. Because of this high incidence, the excessive renal excretion of Ca has been considered to be etiologically important in stone formation. Thus, considerable work has been directed toward the delineation of pathogenesis, diagnostic criteria, and treatment of hypercalciuria.

ROLE OF HYPERCALCIURIA IN STONE FORMATION

The mechanism by which hypercalciuria contributes to Ca stone formation is not totally understood. A recent study indicates that the urinary state of saturation (activity product ratio, APR) with respect to brushite and Ca oxalate is directly correlated with the urinary Ca concentration (Figures 9 and 10).[4,5] Provided the total urine output is not increased, patients with hypercalciuria are more likely than subjects with normocalciuria to pass urine supersaturated with respect to brushite and Ca oxalate [see Figures 4 and 5 (Chapter 2)]. From such a supersaturated environment, the nidi of calcium phosphate and Ca oxalate might be more likely to form and grow.

Two other factors may contribute to the urinary supersatura-

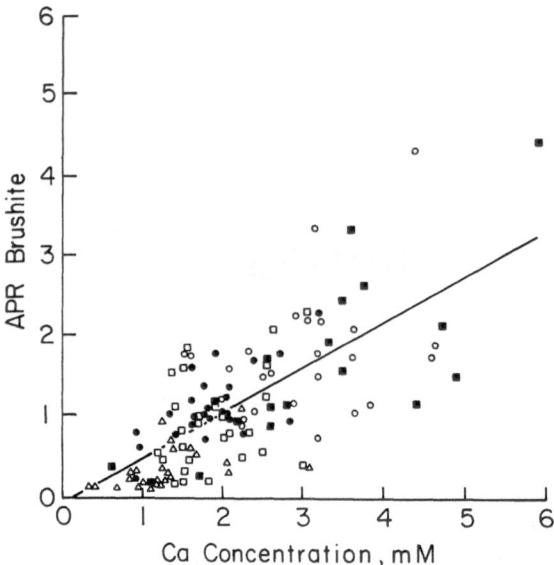

FIGURE 9. Relationship between activity product ratio (APR) of brushite and urinary Ca concentration. An APR value of 1 indicates saturation; greater than 1, supersaturation; and less than 1, undersaturation. The diagonal line represents the regression line ($r = 0.71$). ($\triangle$) Control group; ($\bigcirc$) absorptive hypercalciuria Type I; ($\bullet$) absorptive hypercalciuria Type II; ($\square$) normocalciuric nephrolithiasis; ($\blacksquare$) primary hyperparathyroidism.

tion with respect to Ca salts. In certain patients with primary hyperparathyroidism, urinary pH may be high.[6,7] The APR of brushite may be increased because more of the phosphate would be in the divalent form. Moreover, in patients with hypercalciuria who have an intestinal hyperabsorption of Ca, urinary oxalate may be higher than in normal subjects maintained on the same diet,[8] probably because less Ca may be left in the lumen to complex oxalate. This increase in renal oxalate excretion may contribute to the elevation in urinary APR of Ca oxalate encountered in patients with hypercalciuria.

The scheme outlined above is not the sole cause of stone formation, since many subjects do not form stones, despite hypercalciuria. Many normal subjects without stones may have hypercalciuria or pass urine of high Ca concentration because of restricted fluid intake. Renal stones rarely form in patients with hypercalciuria secondary to thyrotoxicosis, sarcoidosis,[9,10] hypercalcemia of malignancy, or treated hypoparathyroidism.[11] Certain patients with primary hyperparathyroidism may not suffer from renal stones despite persistent hypercalciuria.[12] These considerations emphasize the probable operation of other determinants of stone formation, e.g., inhibitors and promoters of crystallization.

The initial work of Howard *et al.*[13] suggested that urine from patients with Ca stones may be lacking or deficient in certain peptides that are potent inhibitors of calcification, as discussed in Chapter 2. This claim was later retracted.[14] Although the renal excretion of some of the inhibitors—such as magnesium,[15] citrate,[16] zinc,[17] and acid mucopolysaccharide[18]—is probably not altered, that of others, such as pyrophosphate,[19] may be deficient in patients with renal stones. There may be other urinary inhibitors

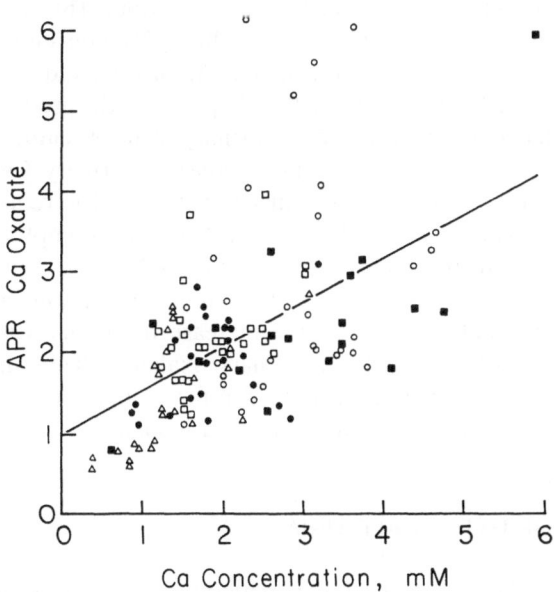

FIGURE 10. Relationship between activity product ratio (APR) of Ca oxalate and urinary Ca concentration ($r = 0.55$). Symbols as in Figure 9.

(e.g., substance "I")[14]; however, their characterization or quantitation has not yet been accomplished.

A recent study[5] suggests the presence in urine of promoters of spontaneous nucleation of calcium phosphate and Ca oxalate. As discussed in Chapter 2, the formation product ratios (FPRs) of brushite and Ca oxalate in the urine of many patients with renal stones were below those obtained in synthetic solutions. The results suggested the presence in the urine of some patients with renal stones of *promoters* of nucleation of Ca phosphate and Ca oxalate. The nature of the promoter(s) has not yet been determined.

The etiological role of hypercalciuria in stone formation has been questioned on other grounds. First, it has been argued that high concentrations of Ca may not render urine supersaturated with respect to Ca oxalate because of the formation of soluble complexes of Ca.[20] Because of an increase in the amount of soluble complexes, the concentration of ionized Ca may not increase significantly despite a high total Ca concentration. This problem is encountered, however, only at very high Ca concentrations of greater than 400 mg/liter, a range seldom encountered in patients. Second, it has been suggested that hypercalciuria produced by a high-Ca diet may not increase the urinary state of saturation with respect to Ca oxalate, because the increase in urinary Ca may be compensated by a decrease in urinary oxalate.[21] The reduced oxalate excretion was assumed to occur from the complexation of oxalate by Ca in the intestinal tract.[22] Many patients with hypercalciuria, however, have an intestinal hyperabsorption of Ca.[3,23] Following an oral load of Ca, the increase in urinary Ca is more prominent than the reduction in urinary oxalate.[24] Thus, hypercalciuria is usually associated with a significant increase in the urinary state of saturation with respect to Ca oxalate.

CAUSES OF HYPERCALCIURIA

Three major causes of hypercalciuria, each associated with nephrolithiasis, have been recognized.[1,3,25,26] Resorptive hypercalciuria, which is characterized by primary hyperparathyroidism, will be discussed in detail in Chapter 4. The initial event is the excessive resorption of bone from the hypersecretion of parathyroid hormone (PTH) by abnormal parathyroid tissue (Figure 11a). The intestinal absorption of Ca may be elevated.[1,3,23] These effects increase the circulating concentration of Ca and the renal filtered

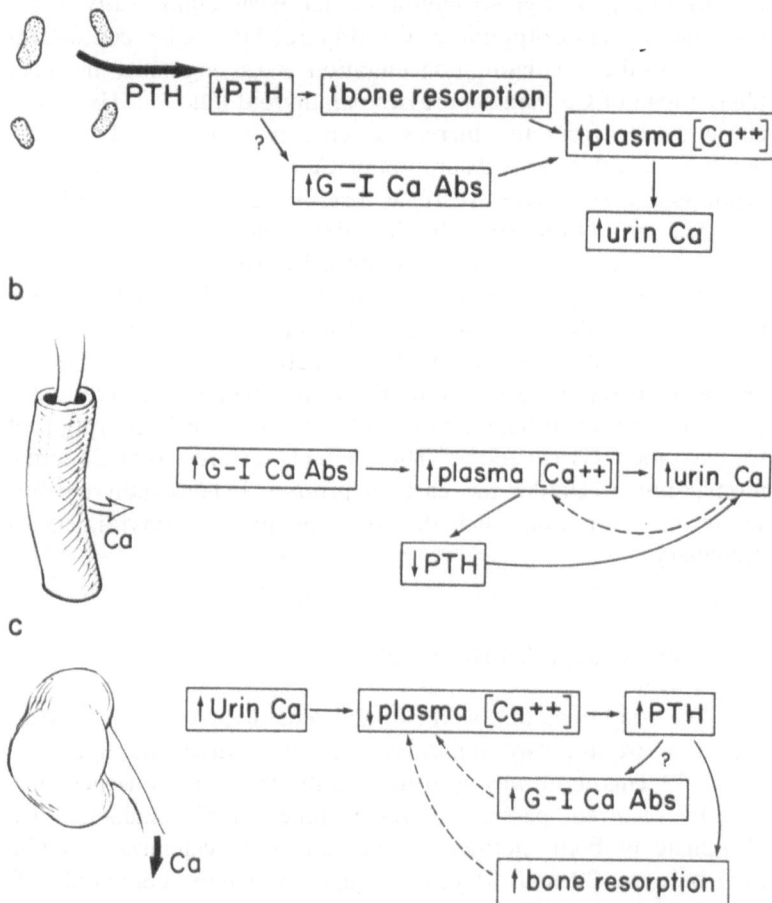

FIGURE 11. Scheme for (a) resorptive hypercalciuria (primary hyperparathyroidism), (b) absorptive hypercalciuria, and (c) renal hypercalciuria ("renal leak"). (PTH) Parathyroid hormone; (G-I Ca Abs) gastrointestinal Ca absorption; (Urin Ca) urinary Ca.

load of Ca. The occurrence of hypercalciuria in hyperparathyroidism seems paradoxical, since the primary renal action
of PTH is the stimulation of renal tubular reabsorption of Ca.[27]
Hypercalciuria is often encountered in primary hyperparathyroidism, however, because the increase in the renal filtered
load of Ca is usually predominant.

In absorptive hypercalciuria,[3,25] the basic abnormality is the
intestinal hyperabsorption of Ca (Figure 11b). The consequent
increase in the circulating concentration of Ca augments the renal
filtered load of Ca, and suppresses parathyroid function. Hypercalciuria ensues from the increased renal filtered load of Ca and
reduced renal tubular reabsorption of Ca consequent to parathyroid
suppression. The excessive renal loss of Ca compensates for the
high Ca absorption from the intestinal tract and maintains the
serum concentration of Ca in the normal range.

In renal hypercalciuria,[26,28] the primary abnormality is the
impairment in the renal tubular reabsorption of Ca (Figure 11c).
The consequent reduction in the circulating concentration of Ca
stimulates parathyroid function. There may be an excessive mobilization of Ca from bone and an enhanced intestinal absorption of
Ca from the PTH excess.[1,29] These effects restore serum Ca to the
normal range. Unlike the case in primary hyperparathyroidism,
serum Ca is normal and the state of hyperparathyroidism is
secondary.

HISTORICAL CONSIDERATIONS

The conditions of absorptive and renal hypercalciurias probably comprise the two major variants of "idiopathic hypercalciuria."[3] This term was used to describe the condition characterized by recurrent passage of renal stones of Ca oxalate of Ca
phosphate or both, normocalcemia, and hypercalciuria.[30] White
men between 20 and 50 years of age were most commonly affected. The serum P concentration was sometimes reduced, although it remained within the normal range in most patients.[3,9,24,26,31−33] Besides hypercalciuria, the renal excretion of

oxalate has been reported to be slightly elevated,[8] as discussed previously. However, urinary pH and contents of magnesium,[15] citrate,[16] phosphate, sodium, and potassium were found to be indistinguishable from those of control subjects.

In 1953, Albright *et al.*,[34] noting a history of urinary tract infection in some of their patients, suggested that the cause of hypercalciuria was a decreased renal tubular reabsorption of Ca, consequent to pyelonephritis. In 1958, Henneman *et al.*[30] found intestinal hyperabsorption of Ca in some of their patients. This increased absorption was attributed to the "compensatory parathyroid hyperplasia" resulting from "primary renal tubular hypercalciuria."

Subsequently, many conflicting reports have appeared supporting either the primacy of "renal leak" or an intestinal hyperabsorption of Ca for the genesis of hypercalciuria. In support of the renal leak hypothesis, it was shown that urinary Ca remained higher than normal on a low-Ca diet, and that some patients with idiopathic hypercalciuria were in negative Ca balance.[35,36] Moreover, the circulating concentration of immunoreactive PTH was clearly elevated despite normocalcemia in some patients.[26] Other studies, however, have disclosed that hypercalciuria could be corrected by a low-Ca diet or by inhibition of Ca absorption with cellulose phosphate, and that many patients are not in negative Ca balance.[3,37,38] Peacock and Nordin[39] found that the tubular reabsorption and renal threshold of calcium in patients with hypercalciuria were the same as those with normal urinary Ca, and disputed that a renal leak of Ca was present. Finn *et al.*[40] studied a man who received a kidney from his father, who had idiopathic hypercalciuria. Since the son did not develop hypercalciuria, the excessive renal excretion of Ca in the father was not believed to be renal in origin.

It has therefore been suggested that the primary abnormality in at least some patients with idiopathic hypercalciuria may be the intestinal hyperabsorption of Ca.[3,25] Hyperabsorption of Ca has been found in idiopathic hypercalciuria by several independent techniques. During the fasting state, when absorbed Ca does not contribute significantly to urinary Ca, the renal Ca excretion was found to be normal,[25,28] a finding that indicated that the renal handling of Ca was not defective. Following an oral load of Ca, the increase in urinary Ca excretion was exaggerated, a result that suggested that Ca was absorbed excessively from the intestinal tract.[28] Moreover, parathyroid function as measured by renal excretion of cyclic AMP (cAMP) and serum immunoreactive PTH (iPTH) was normal or suppressed, and became more suppressed with an oral Ca load.[3]

These apparently conflicting results could be resolved if it is assumed that idiopathic hypercalciuria is comprised of two separate entities—renal hypercalciuria[26,28] and absorptive hypercalciuria.[3,25] The existence of the two conditions can no longer be disputed. The prevailing disagreement is a relatively minor one, and concerns the apparent variation in the relative incidence of the two conditions. Thus, in a series of Coe et al.,[26] a majority of patients with idiopathic hypercalciuria had renal hypercalciuria; a third probably had absorptive hypercalciuria, since they had normal parathyroid function. Other reports had indicated a preponderance of those with absorptive hypercalciuria.[3,25]

DIAGNOSTIC CRITERIA FOR HYPERCALCIURIAS

A reliable method for the differentiation of the three forms of hypercalciuria has been developed.[3] An important feature of this technique is a constant dietary regimen by which various dietary influences on renal excretion of Ca[3,41–44] were carefully controlled. While the patients were maintained on a constant liquid synthetic diet (Calcitest, Doyle Pharmaceutical Co.), containing 400 mg Ca, 800 mg P, and 100 meq Na/day, accurate measures of parathyroid function, intestinal Ca absorption, and Ca metabolism were obtained simultaneously. These studies have unequivocally demonstrated the existence of absorptive and renal hypercalciurias and permitted a formulation of diagnostic criteria for these variants of idiopathic hypercalciuria as well as for primary hyperparathyroidism (Table III). Since primary hyperparathyroidism will be discussed in Chapter 4, its features will be presented

TABLE III. Diagnostic Criteria for Hypercalciurias

Criterion[a]	PHPT[a]	AH-I[a]	AH-II[a]	AH-III[a]	RH[a]
Serum Ca	↑	N	N	N	N
Serum P	↓/N	N	N	↓	N
Urinary Ca[b]	↑/N	↑	N	↑/N	↑
Serum iPTH	↑	N/↓	N/↓	N/↓	↑
Urinary cAMP[b]	↑	N/↓	N/↓	N/↓	↑
Urinary cAMP (fasting)	↑	N	N	N	↑
Urinary cAMP (1 g Ca load)	↑	N	N	N	N
α (100 mg Ca)	↑/N	↑	↑/N	↑/N	↑/N
Urinary Ca (1 g Ca load)	↑/N	↑	↑	↑	↑/N
Urinary Ca (fasting)	↑/N	N	N	N	↑
Bone density	N/↓	N	N	N	N/↓

[a](AH-I, -II, -III) Absorptive hypercalciuria, Types I, II, and III; (cAMP) cyclic AMP; (iPTH) immunoreactive parathyroid hormone; (PHPT) primary hyperparathyroidism; (RH) renal hypercalciuria; (↑) high; (↓) low; (N) normal.
[b]24-Hour urinary values on a low-Ca diet of 400 mg Ca/day. Fasting samples represent 2-hr urine collections obtained in the morning following an overnight fast.[28] "One-g Ca load" samples were obtained over a 4-hr period subsequent to an oral ingestion of 1 g Ca. Fractional Ca absorption (α) was obtained from fecal recovery of radioactivity following oral administration of radiocalcium with 100 mg Ca.[23] Bone density was obtained in the distal third of the radius by photon absorptiometry.[3]

mainly as a source of comparison with absorptive and renal hypercalciurias. Absorptive hypercalciuria consisted of three types.[1,5,32] In absorptive hypercalciuria Type I (AH-I), there was an excessive renal excretion of Ca at all levels of Ca intake,[3] a finding suggesting a hyperabsorptive state independent of Ca intake. In absorptive hypercalciuria Type II (AH-II), an enhanced Ca excretion was demonstrated only at a high intake of Ca.[1,5] The results indicated that intestinal Ca absorption was increased at high Ca intake, but may be normal at low intake. In absorptive hypercalciuria Type III (AH-III), or hypophosphatemic absorptive hypercalciuria,[32] the serum concentration of P was low; otherwise, the features were the same as in AH-I or AH-II.

In primary hyperparathyroidism, the serum Ca concentration was elevated in the majority of cases.[1] Even though serum Ca was normal in a minority of cases, hypercalcemia had been found prior to this evaluation in all cases. The serum concentration of P was low in a minority of cases and normal in the majority of cases. Hypercalciuria was encountered in approximately two thirds of cases. In AH-I, AH-II, and renal hypercalciuria, the serum concentrations of Ca and P were within the normal range. Serum Ca was normal, but serum P low, in AH-III. On an intake of 400 mg Ca/day, urinary Ca was elevated, being greater than 200 mg/day, but was less than the intake of 400 mg/day in AH-I; it was normal in AH-II, and high or normal in AH-III. Urinary Ca was high or high normal in renal hypercalciuria.

Parathyroid function was assessed from measurements of urinary cAMP [45,46] and of serum iPTH. Urinary cAMP was measured in 24-hr samples obtained under constant dietary regimen. It was elevated in 67% of cases with primary hyperparathyroidism (>5.4 μmol/g creatinine), and in 44% of cases with renal hypercalciuria.[1] It was normal or low in absorptive hypercalciuria. The results are consistent with the previous demonstration that serum iPTH is often elevated in primary hyperparathyroidism [47,48] and in renal hypercalciuria,[26] and is normal or low in absorptive hypercalciuria.[1,3] Urinary cAMP was usually high in primary hyperparathyroidism and renal hypercalciuria during the fasting state. Whereas it did not change significantly following an oral Ca load of 1 g (as compared with the fasting value) in primary hyperparathyroidism, it generally returned toward normal in renal hypercalciuria.[28] The results are compatible with the suppressibility of PTH secretion by oral Ca load in renal hypercalciuria.

In primary hyperparathyroidism and in secondary hyperparathyroidism of renal hypercalciuria, the intestinal Ca absorption (fractional Ca absorption) from an oral load of 1000 mg was elevated in the majority of cases.[1] Whereas it was invariably high in absorptive hypercalciuria Type I, it was increased in only some of the patients with absorptive hypercalciuria Types II and III. The intestinal Ca absorption from a high Ca load (1000 mg) was estimated from the extent of urinary Ca excretion following oral Ca load. It was often high in primary hyperparathyroidism and renal hypercalciuria, and invariably increased in all three forms of absorptive hypercalciuria.

The state of bone and Ca metabolism was assessed noninvasively from fasting urinary Ca, a comparison of absorbed and urinary Ca, and from bone density (of the radius) by ^{125}I-photon absorptiometry.[3] During the fasting state, urinary Ca may reflect the extent of mobilization of Ca from bone, since there is no significant absorption of Ca from the intestinal tract.[25] In primary hyperparathyroidism and renal hypercalciuria, fasting urinary Ca was usually or invariably high, urinary Ca often exceeded absorbed Ca, and bone density was sometimes reduced. In contrast, these determinations were usually normal in absorptive hypercalciuria. The results suggest that there may be in primary hyperparathyroidism and renal hypercalciuria, an excessive bone resorption or a negative Ca balance, probably from PTH excess, unlike the case in absorptive hypercalciuria, in which bone is "spared."

The studies of "fast and load" formed the basis for a simple test[28] for the diagnosis of renal hypercalciuria and absorptive hypercalciuria (Figure 12). Renal hypercalciuria was characterized by normocalcemia, high fasting urinary Ca and cAMP, and "suppressible" urinary cAMP following an oral Ca load. All three forms of absorptive hypercalciuria had normal fasting urinary Ca and an exaggerated renal excretion of Ca following an oral Ca load. As discussed earlier, normal (24-hr) urinary Ca with a low-Ca diet (400 mg/day) discriminated absorptive hypercalciuria Type II from Type I.

In absorptive hypercalciuria, white adult men were most commonly affected, and recurrent Ca urolithiasis was the only recognizable clinical manifestation. In renal hypercalciuria, the two sexes were equally affected, and bone disease (osteoporosis) as well as Ca urolithiasis may be present. Some patients may give a history of recurrent urinary tract infections, which sometimes preceded the onset of stone disease.

In this classification, absorptive hypercalciuria and renal hypercalciuria were considered to represent a primary disturbance in intestinal Ca absorption or in renal tubular reabsorption of Ca, re-

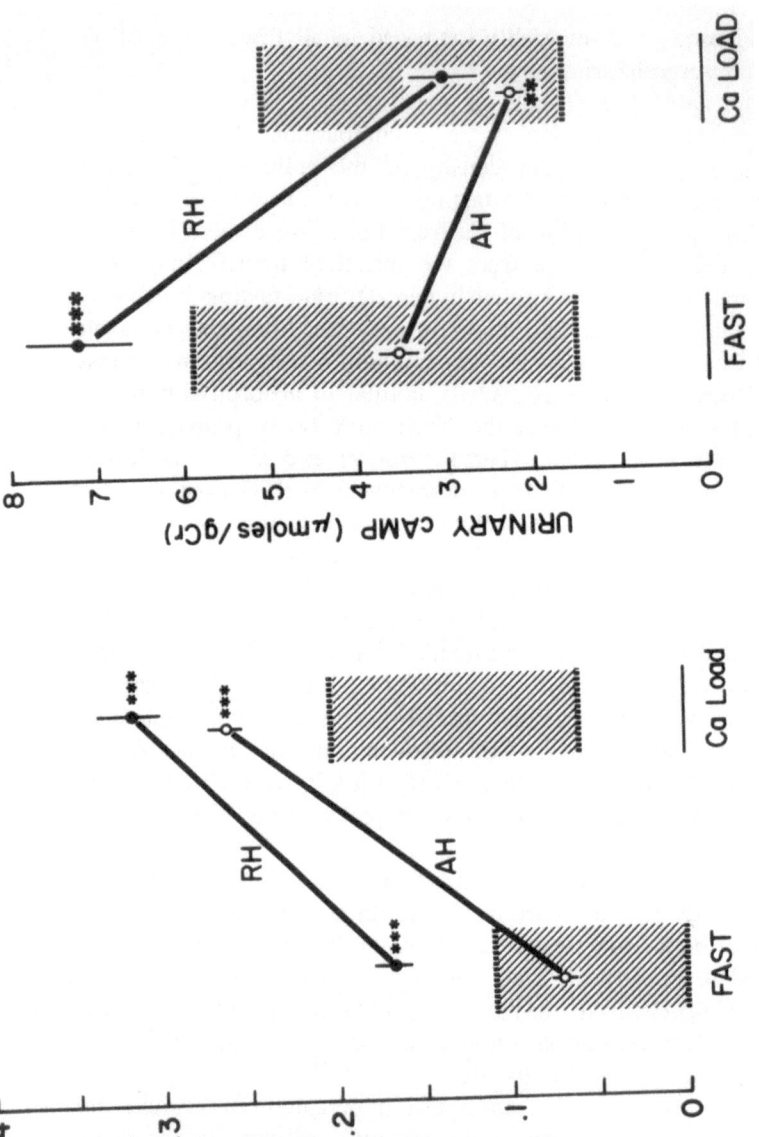

FIGURE 12. Response to fast and oral Ca load (1 g) in renal hypercalciuria (RH) and absorptive hypercalciuria (AH). Urinary Ca and cyclic AMP (cAMP), expressed relative to urinary creatinine (Cr), are shown. The shaded area indicates the range of values in the control group. Values in RH and AH are presented as means ± S.E.M. Significant difference of these values from the control group is denoted by ** for $p < 0.01$ and *** for $p < 0.001$.

spectively. This classification excluded secondary causes, e.g., vitamin D excess or sarcoidosis [49] for the intestinal hyperabsorption of Ca, and renal tubular acidosis [50] and hypoparathyroidism [11] for the renal leak of Ca. In renal hypercalciuria, hypercalciuria may result from several causes, since the primary impairment in the renal tubular reabsorption of Ca may be accompanied by secondary increases in intestinal Ca absorption and in bone resorption. Not all patients with primary hyperparathyroidism suffer from resorptive hypercalciuria; only some have high fasting urinary Ca or are in negative Ca balance.[3] Certain cases with primary hyperparathyroidism may have secondary absorptive hypercalciuria, since their intestinal Ca absorption is elevated.[23,51]

ASSOCIATION WITH HYPERURICOSURIA

Hypercalciuria may be associated with hyperuricosuria. Moreover, certain patients with Ca urolithiasis may present with normocalciuria without any discernible abnormality of Ca metabolism or parathyroid function. These conditions will be discussed in Chapter 5.

GENETICS OF ABSORPTIVE AND RENAL HYPERCALCIURIAS

Many patients with renal or absorptive hypercalciuria may present a rich family history of Ca urolithiasis. However, the exact mode of inheritance is not known. In 1960, McGeown [52] reported that the incidence of stone formation was significantly higher among parents and siblings of patients with renal stones than among relatives of control subjects. In the only other important study involving a large sample population, Resnick et al.[53] reached a similar conclusion for Ca oxalate stones. Their analysis ruled out monogenic inheritance, but suggested an operation of a polygenic system, with a reduced risk for females. They believed that no single biochemical variable could account for the nephrolithiasis.

The study of Resnick *et al.*,[53] however, considered all patients with Ca oxalate stones; it did not attempt to separate them into various etiologies. Since this study was conducted, considerable progress has been made regarding various causes of nephrolithiasis and underlying pathogenetic mechanisms. The genetics of nephrolithiasis should be reinvestigated, utilizing improved diagnostic separation (e.g., among hypercalciurias) and various biochemical derangements as potential "genetic markers."

CLINICAL COURSE

The clinical course of Ca urolithiasis in absorptive and renal hypercalciurias is variable. Ca urolithiasis may begin at any age, though it most commonly begins in young adulthood. In some patients, stone disease may remain active from onset, with persistent formation of new stones. In others, there is some evidence that the stone disease may undergo remission. Certain patients may form no more stones after having formed one. More commonly, particularly in absorptive hypercalciuria, patients may enter long periods of remission between stone episodes, especially during young adult life.

It is interesting to speculate that during the period of clinical remission, various biochemical abnormalities in urine,[5,14,18] typically found in patients with active stone formation, may be lost or become less apparent. A total loss of these abnormalities would favor the operation of environmental rather than genetic factors for the pathogenesis of absorptive and renal hypercalciurias. The utilization of newly developed physicochemical and diagnostic techniques described earlier should help resolve this question.

CAUSES OF THE INTESTINAL HYPERABSORPTION OF CALCIUM

The intestinal absorption of Ca is frequently elevated in primary hyperparathyroidism[3,23] and in renal hypercalciuria,[28,29] and is invariably increased in absorptive hypercalciuria,[3] as shown previously. Because of the well-known action of vitamin D in stimulating intestinal Ca absorption, the pathogenetic role of vitamin D was sought.[51]

In states of hyperparathyroidism (primary hyperparathyroidism and renal hypercalciuria), the plasma concentration of $1\alpha,25$-dihydroxycholecalciferol [$1\alpha,25$-(OH)$_2$D] was significantly increased and positively correlated with intestinal Ca absorption (Figure 13).[51] In a preliminary study,[54] treatment of con-

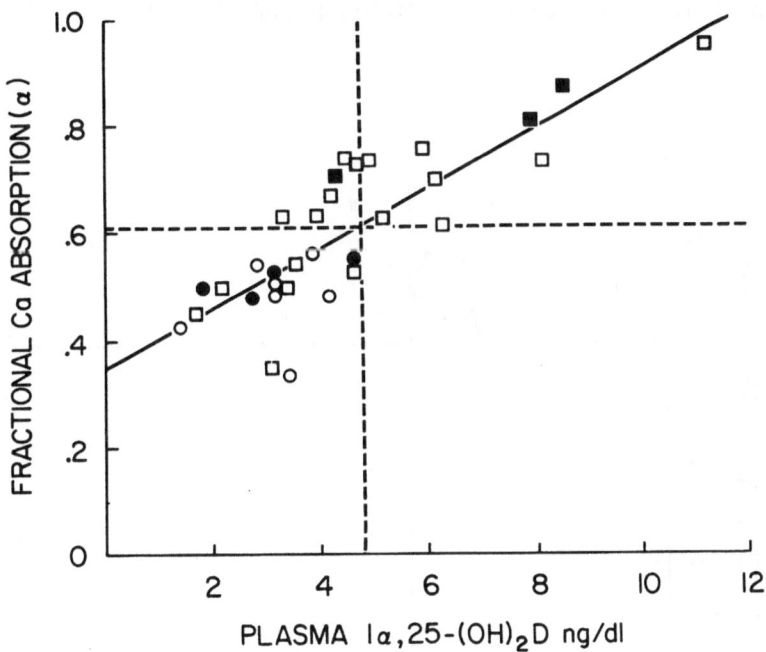

FIGURE 13. Dependence of fractional Ca absorption (α) on plasma concentration of $1\alpha,25$-dihydroxycholecalciferol [$1\alpha,25$-(OH)$_2$D] in primary hyper para-thyroidism (PHPT) and in renal hypercalciuria (RH). The horizontal dashed line indicates the upper range of normal for α; the vertical dashed line represents the upper limit of normal for plasma $1\alpha,25$-(OH)$_2$D. The solid diagonal line represents regression for the combined group of PHPT ($\square$), RH ($\blacksquare$), normocalciuric nephrolithiasis (NN) ($\bullet$), and control ($\bigcirc$) ($r = 0.83$, $p < 0.001$).

trol subjects with crude parathyroid extract significantly raised fractional Ca absorption, commensurate with a rise in plasma concentration of $1\alpha,25\text{-}(OH)_2D$. The results are consistent with studies in experimental animals that demonstrate the capacity of PTH to stimulate the renal synthesis of $1\alpha,25\text{-}(OH)_2D$.[55] Thus, the intestinal hyperabsorption of Ca in primary hyperparathyroidism and renal hypercalciuria is probably the result of PTH-dependent stimulation of the production of $1\alpha,25\text{-}(OH)_2D$.

In absorptive hypercalciuria, the circulating concentration of $1\alpha,25\text{-}(OH)_2D$ is also increased[51] (4.5 ± 1.1 S.D. vs. 3.4 ± 0.9 ng/dl in control subjects, $p < 0.01$) (Figure 14). However, the

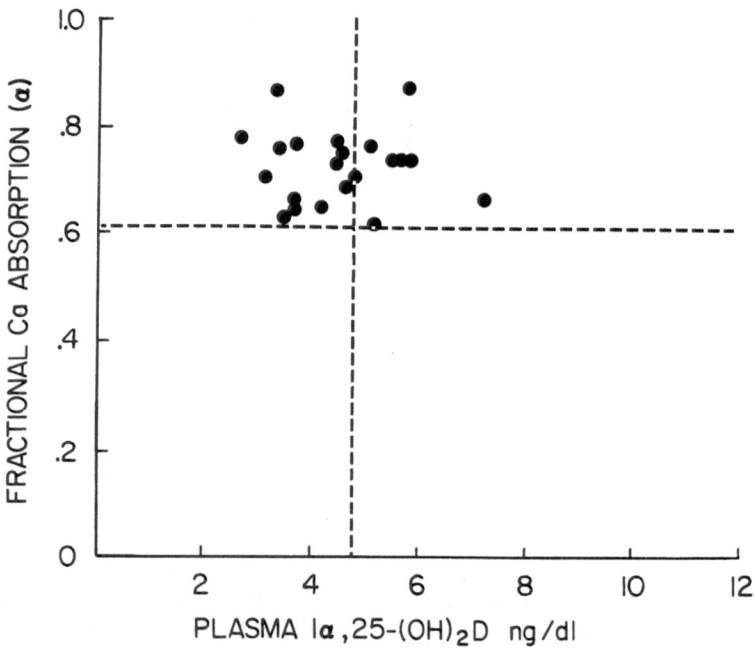

FIGURE 14. Lack of dependence of fractional Ca absorption (α) on plasma concentration of $1\alpha,25$-dihydroxycholecalciferol [$1\alpha,25\text{-}(OH)_2D$] in absorptive hypercalciuria.

plasma concentration of vitamin D metabolite was not correlated with intestinal Ca absorption, and in many cases, the intestinal Ca absorption was inappropriately high for the amount of $1\alpha,25$-$(OH)_2D$ in plasma. The results suggest that the increased circulating concentration of $1\alpha,25$-$(OH)_2D$ may not be the sole cause of the high intestinal Ca absorption. This conclusion is supported by the evidence that thiazide therapy does not restore normal intestinal Ca absorption in absorptive hypercalciuria, whereas it has been shown that it usually reduces intestinal Ca absorption to normal in renal hypercalciuria.[29] Furthermore, treatment with prednisone (50 mg/day for 8 days) does not correct the intestinal hyperabsorption of Ca in absorptive hypercalciuria, whereas it does so in sarcoidosis,[49] in which there is probably a vitamin-D-dependent intestinal Ca hyperabsorption.

The cause for the apparent increased synthesis of $1\alpha,25$-$(OH)_2D$ in absorptive hypercalciuria is not known. Shen et al.[32] also found this increase and attributed it to hypophosphatemia, resulting from an impaired renal tubular reabsorption of phosphate. Although hypophosphatemia has been shown to be an important regulator of $1\alpha,25$-$(OH)_2D$ synthesis in experimental animals,[56] there is currently no evidence for this regulatory role in man. Moreover, the serum concentration of phosphorus may not be low, and was not correlated with the circulating concentration of $1\alpha,25$-$(OH)_2D$ or intestinal Ca absorption.[51] Nevertheless, in those patients with absorptive hypercalciuria who have hypophosphatemia (AH-III), the operation of the phosphate-dependent synthesis of vitamin D metabolite is theoretically possible.

TREATMENT OF HYPERCALCIURIAS

The management of primary hyperparathyroidism will be discussed in Chapter 4. The following discussion summarizes pertinent aspects of physiological action, physicochemical effects, and side effects of current available drugs for Ca urolithiasis (Table IV).

TABLE IV. Mode of Action of Therapeutic Modalities[a]

	Sodium cellulose PO$_4$	Thiazide	Orthophosphate	Diphosphonate
Urinary Ca	↓↓↓	↓↓	↓	—
Urinary P	↑	↑	↑↑↑	—
Urinary Ox	↑↑	↑	↑/—	↑/—
Urinary P$_2$O$_7$	—	↑	↑↑	—
Brushite APR	↓↓	↓	↑	—
FPR	—	↑	↑	↑
CG	—	—	↓/—	↓
Ca Ox APR	↓/—	↓	↓	—
FPR	—	↑	↑	↑
CG	—	—	↓/—	↓
Indications	AH-I	RH	AH-III	

[a] Abbreviations: (↑) increase; (↓) decrease; (—) no change; (Ox) oxalate; (P$_2$O$_7$) pyrophosphate; (APR) activity product ratio; (FPR) formation product ratio; (CG) crystal growth; (AH-I) absorptive hypercalciuria Type I; (RH) renal hypercalciuria; (AH-III) hypophosphatemic absorptive hypercalciuria.

Sodium Cellulose Phosphate

Physiology. This drug represents the treatment of choice for absorptive hypercalciuria. Sodium cellulose phosphate [3,7,38,42,57] is a nonabsorbable ion-exchange resin with a high affinity for Ca^{2+}. The biological activity (Ca binding) is due to the phosphate group, which is covalently bound to cellulose. When it is given orally, dietary and secreted Ca exchanges for sodium in resin; the complex of Ca and cellulose phosphate is excreted in the feces. The drug is customarily given with food two or three times a day. It therefore inhibits intestinal Ca absorption by limiting the amount of Ca available for absorption. It does not alter the basic Ca-transport process.

The goal of therapy with sodium cellulose phosphate in absorptive hypercalciuria is to provide an appropriate amount of the drug to reduce the high intestinal Ca absorption to normal, and not below normal. When this task is accomplished, urinary Ca invariably decreases toward normal. At a dosage of 5 g three times a day, sodium cellulose phosphate typically lowers urinary Ca by 150–200 mg/day.[3,57]

Physical Chemistry. The mechanism of action of sodium cellulose phosphate from the physicochemical standpoint is well established. Treatment is usually accompanied by a slight to moderate increase in urinary phosphorus.[7,42,57] This increase probably reflects the partial hydrolysis of phosphate in the intestinal tract, or stimulation of parathyroid function (toward normal) as the intestinal hyperabsorption of Ca is corrected, or both. The decrease in urinary Ca, however, is much more prominent than the increase in urinary phosphorus.[57] Thus, the urinary APR of brushite (state of saturation) decreases,[7,42,57] usually from supersaturation to undersaturation.

Sodium cellulose phosphate causes a significant increase in renal oxalate excretion.[58,59] This increase is believed to be the result of complexation of Ca in the intestinal lumen by sodium cellulose phosphate. Thus, less oxalate is "bound" to Ca, and more oxalate is available for absorption. When sodium cellulose phosphate is given at a dosage of 5 g three times a day with a low-Ca diet (400 mg Ca/day), urinary oxalate may increase two- to threefold.[58] Urinary Ca, however, declines more prominently or to an equivalent degree. Thus, the urinary APR of Ca oxalate decreases or does not change significantly.[58,59] Despite a significant increase in urinary oxalate, urine specimens do not become more supersaturated with respect to Ca oxalate. On a less restricted Ca diet (500–700 mg Ca/day), sodium cellulose phosphate does not cause as marked an increase in urinary oxalate[59]; urinary oxalate is usually less than 50 mg/day. The decline in urinary Ca, however, is also considerably less. Thus, with both Ca diets, the effect of sodium cellulose phosphate on the urinary APR of Ca oxalate is less dramatic than its effect on the APR of brushite.

Sodium cellulose phosphate apparently does not modify renal excretion of inhibitors of crystallization. No significant change in urinary content of citrate, sulfate, and pyrophosphate has been reported.[57] The treatment does not significantly modify the urinary FPR (limit of metastability) or the crystal growth of brushite or Ca oxalate.[57,58] The results suggest that sodium cellulose phosphate does not produce any change in inhibition of spontaneous nucleation or crystal growth of Ca salts.

Clinical Response. A number of reports have appeared suggesting that sodium cellulose phosphate may be useful in the control of Ca stone formation. Rapado *et al.*[60] gave sodium cellulose phosphate (15 g/day) to 15 patients with idiopathic hypercalciuria. Treatment was followed by a decrease in urinary Ca from a mean of 324 to 149 mg/day, and an increase in urinary phosphorus from a mean of 723 to 927 mg/day. The intestinal Ca absorption decreased in every case. Rose and Harrison[61] treated 24 patients with idiopathic hypercalciuria with sodium cellulose phosphate. Satisfactory long-term control of renal stone formation with sodium cellulose phosphate alone was encountered in 9 of 11 patients; in 2 patients, there was partial but insufficient control with sodium cellulose phosphate alone. In 7 patients, satisfactory long-term control was obtained with sodium cellulose phosphate and thiazide given concurrently. Blacklock and MacLeod[62] gave sodium cellulose phosphate to 9 patients with idiopathic hypercalciuria at a dosage of 15 g/day over a 4-year period. Subjective clinical improvement (decreased incidence of stone passage or surgical operation for stones) was noted in every case. Urinary Ca decreased commensurate with the fall in intestinal Ca absorption.

In our study,[63] the rate of new stone formation was found to decrease during treatment, commensurate with a fall in urinary state of saturation with respect to brushite. This study represents the first instance in which the clinical response has been correlated with objective changes. The selective effect of sodium cellulose phosphate on crystallization of brushite, rather than of Ca oxalate, underscores the importance of brushite in stone formation (see Chapter 2).

Specifically, indications for sodium cellulose phosphate therapy are those patients with AH-I, i.e., patients who present with: (1) recurrent Ca urolithiasis (Ca oxalate, Ca phosphate), (2) absence of bone disease, (3) normocalcemia, (4) fasting urinary $Ca < 0.11$ mg/mg creatinine during 2 hr following an overnight fast,[28] (5) urinary $Ca > 0.20$ mg/mg creatinine during 4 hr following an ingestion of 1 g Ca,[28] (6) urinary $Ca > 200$ mg/day on a diet containing 400 mg Ca and 100 meq sodium/day, and (7) normal serum iPTH or urinary cAMP. In patients with AH-II, calcium restriction may be attempted before proceeding to sodium cellulose phosphate therapy.

The customary dosages are as follows: if urinary $Ca < 300$ mg/day, sodium cellulose phosphate 5 g twice a day with meals and magnesium gluconate 1 g twice a day at bedtime and before breakfast (separately from sodium cellulose phosphate); if urinary $Ca > 300$ mg/day, sodium cellulose phosphate 5 g three times a day with meals and magnesium gluconate 1.5 g twice a day at bedtime and before breakfast. Patients should be continued on a low-Ca diet. Excessive oxalate ingestion should be discouraged.

Side Effects. Few side effects are expected if sodium cellulose phosphate is given only to those with absorptive hypercalciuria and if it is not given in excessive amounts. Parathyroid function, as measured by serum PTH and urinary cAMP, has remained within the normal range.[63] Bone density, determined in the distal third of the radius by ^{125}I-photon absorptiometry, has not changed. Serum concentrations of iron, copper, and zinc, and urinary zinc, have not been altered significantly. Hypomagnesemia and reduced renal excretion of magnesium may develop during treatment with sodium cellulose phosphate, because of binding of magnesium by the resin.[64] They may be avoided, however, by oral magnesium supplementation (1 g magnesium gluconate twice a day, separately from sodium cellulose phosphate).[63]

However, secondary hyperparathyroidism and bone disease may develop if sodium cellulose phosphate is given in excessive amounts, or if it is given to patients with normal intestinal Ca absorption. It is therefore imperative that the diagnosis of absorptive hypercalciuria is clearly established in patients for whom the treatment is to be undertaken. The drug should not be given chronically to those with primary hyperparathyroidism or renal hypercalciuria or to those with normocalciuric nephrolithiasis and normal intestinal Ca absorption. Moreover, urinary Ca and parathyroid function should be monitored closely (every 4–5 months) during treatment, and the dosage of the drug altered accordingly.

Thiazide Diuretic

Physiology. The rationale for the use of thiazide in the treatment of Ca urolithiasis[65] is based on the ability of the drug to reduce renal Ca excretion. Since the initial report of Lamberg and Kuhlback[66] in 1959, numerous reports have appeared showing the efficacy of thiazide in lowering urinary Ca.[26,29,65,67]

The mechanism by which thiazide reduces urinary Ca has been a subject of extensive investigation.[67,68] It is generally agreed that the "hypocalciuric" action of thiazide is principally renal in origin and that it requires extracellular volume depletion and the presence of PTH.[68] When extracellular volume depletion is prevented by administration of a large amount of sodium, thiazide-induced reduction in urinary Ca is largely blunted.[68]

Some of the actions of thiazide simulate those of PTH. Both thiazide[68] and PTH[27] reduce renal Ca excretion (at the same filtered load of Ca) and augment renal excretion of phosphorus,[6,69] pyrophosphate,[69] and zinc.[70,71] There is no convincing evidence, however, that thiazide augments the secretion of PTH or stimulates renal adenyl cyclase.[67] Initial studies suggested that thiazide might cause parathyroid hyperplasia or stimulate bone resorption[72]; however, these studies have not been confirmed. In acute studies in the dog,[73] the hypocalciuric effect of thiazide is lost in the absence of parathyroid glands. This finding has been attributed to the delayed renal excretion of thiazide in parathyroidectomized animals. In man,[74] the renal excretion of thiazide is not dependent on PTH, and thiazide acutely lowers urinary Ca both in control subjects and in patients with hypoparathyroidism. During chronic administration of thiazide, however, the fall in urinary Ca is either absent or less prominent in patients with hypoparathyroidism than in control subjects.[67,68]

Even though the precise mechanism may not be fully understood, thiazide clearly augments renal tubular reabsorption of Ca and lowers urinary Ca. In patients with renal hypercalciuria, it has been shown to correct the renal leak of Ca, restore normal parathyroid function,[26] and "correct" the intestinal hyperabsorption of Ca.[29] It is therefore the drug of choice for renal hypercalciuria.

Physical Chemistry. The mode of action of thiazide from the physicochemical standpoint is partly understood. Thiazide reduces the urinary APRs (state of saturation) of brushite and Ca oxalate in most patients by lowering the urinary concentration of Ca.[69,75]

However, thiazide may augment renal excretion of phosphate and oxalate, and raise pH,[69,75] by a mechanism not fully understood. These effects may "overcome" the effect of a fall in urinary Ca, and probably account for the lack of a significant change in the urinary state of saturation with respect to Ca salts encountered in some patients.[69,75]

Another action of thiazide is the promotion of renal excretion of inhibitors of crystallization, such as magnesium,[69] zinc,[70,71] and pyrophosphate.[69] This drug action probably accounts for the increase in the urinary FPRs of brushite[69] and Ca oxalate,[75] a finding that suggests an inhibition of spontaneous nucleation of these Ca salts. Thiazide probably exerts the same physicochemical effects in patients with renal hypercalciuria as in those with absorptive hypercalciuria.

Clinical Response. Although thiazide is ideally suited for the treatment of renal hypercalciuria from the physiological standpoint,[26,29] it has been used in both renal and absorptive hypercalciuria with good clinical response. The customary dosage is hydrochlorothiazide, 50 mg twice a day, with potassium supplements (40–60 meq/day). Trichloromethiazide (4 mg/day) or chlorthalidone (50 mg/day)[76] may be substituted for hydrochlorothiazide. Hydrochlorothiazide must be given twice a day because of its shorter half-life, whereas others need be given only once daily. The effects of the three drugs on renal Ca excretion are comparable. Although the physicochemical effects on stone formation have been examined only for hydrochlorothiazide, the other two drugs probably exert similar effects.

Side Effects. Side effects include hypokalemia, extra-cellular volume depletion, magnesium depletion, hyperuricemia, and hypercalcemia.[77,78] Without potassium replacement, hypokalemia may develop and cause lethargy, muscle cramping, and weakness. While ingestion of potassium-rich foods may avert this complication, some such foods (e.g., orange juice) may also be high in oxalate content. It is therefore our practice to routinely give potassium supplements (e.g., Slo-K) initially when thiazide therapy is to be initiated. They may be withdrawn subsequently (after 3–6 months). Symptoms of rapid extracellular volume depletion (e.g., dizziness) are usually present during the first few days of thiazide therapy, when the patient sustains a rapid weight loss. It may be prevented by initiating therapy at a lower dose and gradually increasing to full dosage. A significant hypomagnesemia rarely develops during thiazide therapy. It may be overcome by oral magnesium replacement (magnesium gluconate, 1 g, twice a day). In our experience, magnesium therapy may alleviate muscle cramps, especially in the calves, which may appear, albeit rarely, in the absence of hypokalemia. If hyperuricemia is severe (> 10 mg%), allopurinol (300 mg/day) may be required. In most patients, thiazide is well tolerated without significant side effects.

A mild hypercalcemia (up to 10.6 mg%) may ensue during thiazide therapy in normal man.[68] Part of this rise in serum Ca probably reflects the increased protein-bound Ca; the reduction in extracellular fluid volume augments the circulating concentration of proteins and probably causes increased Ca binding. The circulating concentration of ionized Ca is probably also increased from the inhibition of renal Ca loss. The latter mechanism may be predominant in conditions characterized by an excessive skeletal mobilization of Ca, such as primary hyperparathyroidism.[78] Under such circumstances, true hypercalcemia, reflected by a high plasma Ca^{2+} concentration, may be found. These considerations argue against the use of thiazide in resorptive hypercalciuria of primary hyperparathyroidism. When significant hypercalcemia develops (> 11 mg%), thiazide therapy should be stopped and an evaluation for primary hyperparathyroidism initiated.

Recent studies suggest that thiazides may exert long-term effects on bone and Ca metabolism. In patients with renal hypercalciuria, thiazide reduces both the renal excretion of Ca and intestinal Ca absorption.[29] The sequence by which thiazide reduces intestinal Ca absorption may be as follows: decreased urinary Ca→decreased PTH secretion→decreased $1\alpha,25\text{-}(OH)_2D$ synthesis→decreased intestinal Ca absorption. Thus, thiazide may correct compensatory intestinal hyperabsorption of Ca, which results from the primary renal leak of Ca and ensuing secondary hyperparathyroidism. By this means, normal Ca balance may be restored by thiazide therapy. The serum Ca concentration is maintained within the normal range.

In patients with absorptive hypercalciuria, however, thiazide does not significantly alter intestinal Ca absorption, even though it causes an equivalent fall in urinary Ca.[29] Thus, Ca continues to be absorbed excessively even though urinary Ca returns to normal. Thiazide produces these changes, without causing a significant rise in circulating concentration of Ca^{2+}. What is the fate of this "retained" Ca? There are three possible explanations. First, thiazide might promote secretion of Ca into the intestinal lumen. Even though the amount of absorbed Ca (unidirectional uptake from lumen to blood, which was measured in the study cited above) may not have changed, the net Ca absorption may have decreased by a rise in secreted Ca. Thus, Ca balance may be maintained.

If this mechanism is operative in absorptive hypercalciuria, it must also apply to renal hypercalciuria. If so, the Ca balance may become more negative from reduced intestinal Ca absorption and increased secretion in renal hypercalciuria. However, the correction of secondary hyperparathyroidism by thiazide therapy is inconsistent with this hypothesis. If thiazide stimulated intestinal secretion of Ca, the ensuing negative Ca balance would have maintained the state of parathyroid stimulation.

Second, the "retained" Ca might be removed from the circulation by deposition in soft tissues. There is no evidence, however, that thiazide promotes soft-tissue calcification. An increase in serum amylase has been reported during thiazide therapy.[79] This chemical abnormality occurs uncommonly and may not indicate pancreatitis consequent to soft tissue calcification.

Finally, thiazide might promote retention of Ca by bone. Although direct confirmatory experimental evidence is lacking, there is some indirect evidence supporting this hypothesis. Forland et al.[80] found that in patients with primary hyperparathyroidism who had been taking thiazide, the density of the phalanx of the hand measured by ^{125}I-photon absorptiometry was not as depressed as in those who had not been taking thiazide. This study suggests that thiazide might protect bone from the PTH-stimulated bone resorption. In absorptive hypercalciuria, however, parathyroid function may already be suppressed from the increased Ca absorption. Thus, little change would be expected from the further inhibition of PTH action by thiazide. A critical argument against the retention of Ca in bone is the lack of evidence for the development of osteosclerosis or an increase in bone density during chronic thia-zide therapy. If the reduced renal Ca excretion is expressed as bone accretion, a retention of 100 mg Ca/day might be expected during treatment. At that rate, a 37% increase in the Ca content of bone could have occurred in 10 years of thiazide therapy, a change that should have been detected roentgenologically.

Currently, the exact fate of retained Ca during thiazide therapy in absorptive hypercalciuria and renal hypercalciuria is unresolved.

Orthophosphate

Physiology. The rationale for the use of oral orthophosphate for Ca urolithiasis originally was the demonstration by Howard *et al.*[13] that the urine of patients who had been taking orthophosphate lost its ability to calcify rachitic cartilage; i.e., orthophosphate converted "evil" urine to "good" urine. Later, Fleisch *et al.*[81] found that orthophosphate therapy promotes renal excretion of pyrophosphate. However, only part of the inhibition of calcification produced by orthophosphate could be accounted for by the increased pyrophosphate excretion. Although orthophosphate is extensively used today, its mode of action is poorly understood.

Unlike sodium cellulose phosphate, which is nonabsorbable, the sodium and potassium salts of orthophosphate may be absorbed from the intestinal tract by virtue of their high solubility. When given orally, it raises serum phosphorus concentration[82] (acutely) and markedly increases urinary phosphate.[7,42] The orthophosphate therapy may lower urinary Ca by the following mechanism: The rise in serum phosphorus concentration is associated with a reciprocal fall in serum concentration of total and ionized Ca.[82] The latter provides a stimulus to PTH secretion. The serum Ca concentration is restored to the initial value by parathyroid action. The urinary Ca declines, probably consequent to the decrease in the renal filtered load of Ca (at least during initial period), and to the PTH stimulation of the renal tubular reabsorption of Ca. However, parathyroid stimulation has not been found universally during orthophosphate therapy.[83]

The exact mechanism by which orthophosphate lowers serum Ca concentration is uncertain. First, the decrease in serum Ca has been attributed to the rise in serum phosphorus concentration, by implicating the maintenance of a constant $Ca \times P$ product. As will be discussed in Chapter 4, however, such a product has no physicochemical reality. Second, it has been suggested that a rise in serum phosphorus concentration might lower serum Ca concentration by altering Ca transport at the ionic barrier separating interstitial fluid of bone from the extracellular fluid, or by directly inhibiting bone resorption or promoting bone formation.[84]

Third, orthophosphate therapy might reduce serum Ca concentration by inhibiting intestinal Ca absorption. If the regulation of $1\alpha,25$-$(OH)_2D$ synthesis by serum phosphorus concentration is operative,[32,56] there should be a reduced circulating concentration of the vitamin D metabolite, and hence a low intestinal Ca absorption, as the serum phosphorus concentration is increased by orthophosphate therapy. However, the rapid reciprocal change in serum Ca concentration,[82] occurring within minutes of orthophosphate administration in the absence of food, argues against this hypothesis. Nevertheless, a long-term effect of orthophosphate therapy involving vitamin D metabolism cannot be excluded. Thus, in patients with hypophosphatemic absorptive hypercalciuria (AH-III), it is theoretically possible that the intestinal Ca absorption may decrease from the reduced synthesis of $1\alpha,25$-$(OH)_2D$ as the serum P increases during long-term phosphate therapy. Moreover, orthophosphate may inhibit Ca absorption independently of vitamin D metabolism, by direct complexation of Ca. Unfortunately, available data pertaining to the effect of orthophosphate on intestinal Ca absorption are conflicting and do not shed light as to what mechanism might be operative.

Finally, orthophosphate therapy might reduce serum Ca concentration by promoting soft-tissue calcification. Spaulding and

Walser[85] found an increase in the Ca content of soft tissues, particularly of the kidneys, after long-term treatment with orthophosphate in laboratory animals. In man, a deterioration of renal function and calcification of aorta, conjunctiva, heart, and kidneys have been reported during orthophosphate therapy.[86] While this complication occurs more commonly in patients with hypercalcemia, it has also occurred in patients with normocalcemia, in whom the increase in the $Ca \times P$ product in plasma is not excessive.[86] The cause for the soft-tissue calcification remains obscure.

Physical Chemistry. The physicochemical effects of orthophosphate therapy on stone formation are partly understood. It increases the urinary APR of brushite,[7,42] owing to the marked increase in urinary phosphate, and a comparatively less prominent decrease in urinary Ca. It usually decreases the urinary state of saturation with respect to Ca oxalate,[87] because even though urinary oxalate may increase slightly, the decrease in urinary Ca is more prominent. Moreover, orthophosphate promotes renal excretion of pyrophosphate,[42,81] and frequently increases the FPR to brushite[42] and Ca oxalate.[87] It is not known whether this inhibition of the spontaneous nucleation of brushite and Ca oxalate is the result solely of the pyrophosphate action. In certain patients, particularly those with urinary tract infection, orthophosphate may fail to augment the urinary content of pyrophosphate, probably because of the action of bacterial pyrophosphatase. In these patients, there is frequently no change in the FPR of Ca salts.

In summary, orthophosphate probably inhibits stone formation by rendering the urine less saturated with respect to Ca oxalate, and by inhibiting the formation of the nidi of brushite and Ca oxalate. Even though urine may become more supersaturated with respect to brushite, the formation of the brushite nidus is not promoted ordinarily because of the commensurate rise in the limit of metastability (FPR). In the presence of urinary tract infection with reduced pyrophosphate excretion, however, the nidation and subsequent crystal growth of Ca phosphate may be promoted.

Clinical Response. Orthophosphate has been used for the treatment of "idiopathic hypercalciuria."[13,83,86,88–90] The clinical response to orthophosphate has been variable. Some found it to be very effective in preventing new stone formation,[83,88] while others reported its failure to significantly alter the rate of stone passage.[90] As discussed before, orthophosphate therapy is ineffective or may aggravate stone formation in patients with significant urinary tract infection. It may prove to be the treatment of choice for hypophosphatemic absorptive hypercalciuria (AH-III). The customary dosage is 500 mg phosphorus, as the neutral phosphate salt of sodium or potassium, given three or four times daily.

Side Effects. Side effects include nausea, abdominal cramping, and diarrhea. These complications are not serious, however, and may disappear spontaneously or may be overcome by beginning treatment at a lower dosage, and gradually reaching full dosage. Potentially more serious side effects include soft-tissue calcification[86] and parathyroid stimulation,[82,91] as discussed above. Moreover, there is some evidence that orthophosphate therapy may induce bone loss.[91,92] Orthophosphate is contraindicated in patients with renal disease, primary hyperparathyroidism, and urinary tract infection.

Diphosphonate

Physiology. Diphosphonate is a synthetic analogue of pyrophosphate.[93] Unlike pyrophosphate, it is not hydrolyzed *in vivo*. Approximately 5–10% of the oral dose of diphosphonate is absorbed.[94] After "saturation" of bone, the absorbed diphosphonate appears in urine in an unaltered form. Following an oral administration of disodium ethane-1-hydroxy-1,1-diphosphonate (EHDP) at a dosage of 5–20 mg P/kg body weight daily, a sufficient amount of diphosphonate may appear in urine to modify Ca stone formation.[95] Diphosphonate may augment renal tubular reabsorption of phosphate and cause hyperphosphatemia.[96] The intestinal Ca absorption or the plasma concentration of $1\alpha,25\text{-}(OH)_2D$ is not significantly altered,[97] although at a much higher dosage, reduced synthesis of the vitamin D metabolite has been reported in experimental animals.[98]

Physical Chemistry. Most of the studies have been performed with EHDP. When diphosphonate is added to urine or synthetic media *in vitro,* it has been shown to exert inhibition at virtually every step of stone formation. It prevents the formation of the nidus, since the FPRs of brushite[99] and Ca oxalate[100,101] are increased. It retards the growth of nidus, since the rates of crystal growth and aggregation are slowed.[99,101,102] Finally, diphosphonate probably prevents mixed stone formation, since it inhibits heterogeneous nucleation of Ca oxalate by hydroxyapatite or monosodium urate[103] and retards phase transformation of brushite to hydroxyapatite.[104] When EHDP is given to patients with Ca urolithiasis, the only consistent effect produced in urine is an inhibition of crystal growth of brushite and Ca oxalate.[95,105]

Clinical Response. Over a longer period of treatment, EHDP may be useful in preventing new stone formation, particularly in those without preexisting stones.[105] The existing stones may appear less radioopaque and may be more easily passed.

Side Effects. A serious potential complication of diphosphonate is its adverse effect on bone metabolism. It may produce osteomalacia by inhibiting matrix mineralization.[106] Increased osteoid has been found on histological examination of bone. Muscle weakness and a rise in serum alkaline phosphate may herald the development of osteomalacia.[105] Unlike classic forms of osteomalacia, the osteomalacia resulting from diphosphonate therapy is not associated with parathyroid stimulation or hypophosphatemia. This complication limits the usefulness of diphosphonate for Ca urolithiasis.

Magnesium

The interest in the role of magnesium in stone formation stems from the finding that magnesium is an inhibitor of calcification,[107,108] albeit not as effective as pyrophosphate. When magnesium (up to 250 mg/liter) is added to synthetic medium *in vitro,* it increases the FPR of Ca oxalate and the apparent solubility of Ca oxalate.[109] Thus, it may inhibit spontaneous nucleation of Ca oxalate and reduce the state of saturation with respect to Ca oxalate. Another rationale for the use of oral magnesium is based on the contention that it might inhibit intestinal oxalate absorption.[110]

The consequent fall in urinary oxalate would then retard stone formation by lowering the urinary APR of Ca oxalate.

Unfortunately, effects of magnesium therapy on renal oxalate excretion have been variable.[110-112] Moreover, urinary Ca has been shown to increase during oral magnesium therapy,[110,113] a finding that may in part reflect the promotion of Ca–Mg exchange in bone.[114,115] Preliminary studies indicate that oral magnesium therapy in patients with Ca urolithiasis does not produce significant changes in the crystallization of Ca oxalate in urine.[109]

Dietary Restriction

As discussed before,[24] oral Ca load augments the urinary state of saturation with respect to brushite and Ca oxalate in patients with an intestinal hyperabsorption of Ca. Since intestinal Ca absorption is frequently or invariably elevated,[3,23,29] it is advisable to restrict dietary Ca intake in all three forms of hypercalciurias. A very rigid low-Ca diet is not advisable, since it may discourage adherence and may adversely affect general nutrition. A suitable diet, which is reasonably well tolerated, might consist of restriction of milk and all dairy products, and certain other Ca-rich foods, such as molasses and canned whole fish. Moderate amounts of leafy vegetables and fruit juices are allowed because of their nutritional value or fluid load or both, despite high oxalate content.

Oxalate restriction is confined to those foods with high oxalate content that could be omitted or limited from the diet without adversely affecting nutrition or reducing compliance. These foods include chocolate, rhubarb, and tea (drunk alone without food). This recommendation is not meant to disparage the importance of urinary oxalate in stone formation. Reduction in urinary oxalate might be just as effective as that of urinary Ca in reducing the state of saturation with respect to Ca oxalate. Rigid dietary oxalate restriction is not advisable, however, since it is difficult to follow, and since it may not substantially reduce renal oxalate excretion. Oxalate absorption from the diet may be limited because of complexation of oxalate by divalent cations contained in food. Tea drunk during meals, for example, may not significantly alter renal oxalate excretion, whereas it might increase urinary oxalate content when drunk alone.

Fluids

Oral fluid intake may influence stone formation by affecting urine volume. A high urine volume may inhibit stone formation, since it reduces the APR (state of saturation) of Ca salts in urine by diluting ionic constituents of stones. Opposing this action is the dilution of inhibitors, e.g., pyrophosphate, with consequent decline in inhibitory activity, reflected as facilitation of nucleation, crystal growth, and aggregation of Ca salts in urine.

However, a high fluid intake is recommended for the following reasons: First, a fluid load is highly efficient in reducing the urinary APR of Ca salts. A twofold increase in urine volume may reduce urinary activity product ratio by one third to one fourth, since it lowers the activity of both cationic and anionic constituents.[116] Second, an undersaturation or metastable supersaturation with respect to brushite and Ca oxalate can be achieved with a high fluid intake and appropriate medical regimen [63,75] Under such circumstances, a loss of inhibitory activity would have no relevance. Finally, a high urine output might dilute promoters of nucleation and may actually cause an inhibition of nucleation of brushite and Ca oxalate in urine.

The desired goal is to force a sufficient amount of fluids to achieve a urine output of at least 2 liters per day. Under normal conditions, adult patients need to drink approximately ten 10-oz glassfuls of fluid (or 3 quarts) daily to produce 2 liters of urine per day. More fluid must be drunk if patients perspire excessively or do heavy manual work. To avoid "wide fluctuations" of urinary concentration, fluids should be distributed evenly during the day, and 30–60 oz should be drunk at bedtime.

Virtually all forms of fluids are allowed, except for milk or items containing dairy products and excessive amounts of tea (drunk alone). Beer and wine may be drunk, even by those with hyperuricosuria in whom high urinary uric acid content is believed to cause or contribute to Ca stone formation (see Chapter 5) if such patients are receiving allopurinol therapy. Certain fluids may contain substances that, if excreted in urine, might promote stone formation. This potentially adverse effect is usually far outweighed, however, by the beneficial effects of increased urine volume.

"HARMFUL" DRUGS

Certain drugs may aggravate Ca urolithiasis.

Ascorbic acid (vitamin C) has been recommended for the therapy of Ca urolithiasis because of its potential ability to lower urinary pH and enhance the antibacterial activity of other drugs.[117-119] In addition, it has recently become popular to administer ascorbic acid as prophylaxis for the common cold.[120] To date, limited data have appeared to substantiate the value of ascorbic acid either to lower urinary pH in patients with chronic infection or to prevent the development of the common cold.[121-123] Moreover, treatment with ascorbic acid (>2 g/day) has been shown to augment the renal excretion of Ca and oxalate.[124-127] The increased oxalate excretion is believed to be the result of the metabolic conversion of ascorbic acid to oxalate. Although the effect of ascorbic acid therapy on the crystallization of Ca salts has not been examined, this treatment will probably augment urinary saturation with respect to Ca oxalate. High dosages of ascorbic acid should be avoided in patients with Ca urolithiasis.

Oral sodium[43] and nonabsorbable phosphate-binding antacids[41] (e.g., carbonates or silicates of magnesium or aluminum) may increase renal Ca excretion. Despite increased Ca excretion, there is no evidence that these treatments augment the urinary APR (state of saturation) of Ca salts. During sodium load, the rise in urinary sodium increases the ionic strength and decreases the activity coefficient of Ca^{2+}. Thus, the activity of Ca^{2+} may not increase even though the total Ca concentration may be higher.[128] Moreover, antacid therapy reduces phosphate excretion, and may lower the activity of HPO_4^{2-}. This action may compensate for the increased renal Ca excretion. These results suggest that sodium- or phosphate-binding antacids may not be harmful in Ca urolithiasis.

However, the possibility that sodium load might increase the urinary APR of monosodium urate and aggravate stone disease has not been excluded (Chapter 5).

As discussed above, vitamin D may play an important role in the mediation of intestinal hyperabsorption of Ca found in many patients with hypercalciuria.[51] It is unlikely, however, that the amount of vitamin D present in the usual diet or in multivitamin preparations is sufficient to significantly alter the vitamin D metabolism in patients with hypercalciuria.

RATIONAL BASIS FOR THERAPY OF HYPERCALCIURIAS

An ideal form of therapy is one that corrects the specific underlying disorder. This goal is beginning to be realized as the pathogenetic mechanism for the various forms of hypercalciurias and the mode of action of drugs to treat them are being delineated. Tentative criteria for optimum therapy for various causes of hypercalciurias will be presented in Chapter 7.

FUTURE RESEARCH IN HYPERCALCIURIAS

Much research remains to be performed in hypercalciurias. First, the chemical nature and the physiological role of the promoter of spontaneous nucleation needs to be elucidated. This clarification would greatly enhance our current understanding of the pathogenesis of stone formation. Second, the cause of the intestinal hyperabsorption of Ca in hypercalciurias needs to be better appreciated. In particular, the role of vitamin D metabolism needs to be more precisely determined. Third, improved forms of therapy should be sought, including: (1) effective medical treatment for nephrolithiasis of primary hyperparathyroidism and (2) treatment that directly interferes with intestinal Ca transport. Finally, the mode of action and potential hazards of current treatment modalities should be better elucidated.

REFERENCES

1. Pak, C. Y. C., Barilla, D., Bone, H., and Northcutt, C. 1977. Medical management of renal calculi. In *New Concepts in Endocrinology and Metabolism.* L. I. Rose and R. L. Levine, Eds. Grune and Stratton, New York, pp. 97–106.
2. Hodgkinson, A., and Pyrah, L. N. 1958. The urinary calcium and inorganic phosphate in 344 patients with calcium stone of renal origin. *Br. J. Surg.* **46:**10–18.
3. Pak, C. Y. C., Ohata, M., Lawrence, E. C., and Snyder, W. 1974. The hypercalciurias: Causes, parathyroid functions and diagnostic criteria. *J. Clin. Invest.* **54:**387–400.
4. Pak, C. Y. C. 1969. Physiochemical basis for the formation of renal stones of calcium phosphate origin: Calculation of the degree of saturation of urine with respect to brushite. *J. Clin. Invest.* **48:**1914–1922.
5. Pak, C. Y. C., and Holt, K. 1976. Nucleation and growth of brushite and calcium oxalate in urine of stone-formers. *Metabolism* **25:**665–673.
6. Czekalski, S., Loreau, N., Paillard, F., Ardaillou, R., Fillastre, J.-P., and Mallet, E. 1974. Effect of bovine parathyroid hormone 1–34 fragment on renal production and excretion of adenosine 3′,5′ monophosphate in man. *Eur. J. Clin. Invest.* **4:**85–92.
7. Pak, C. Y. C., Cox, J. W., Powell, E., and Bartter, F. C. 1971. Effect of the oral administration of ammonium chloride, sodium phosphate, cellulose phosphate and parathyroid extract on the activity product of brushite in urine. *Am. J. Med.* **50:**67–76.
8. Robertson, W. G., Peacock, M., and Nordin, B. E. C. 1971. Calcium oxalate crystalluria and urine saturation in recurrent renal stone-formers. *Clin. Sci.* **40:**365–374.
9. Parfitt, A. M., Higgins, B. A., Nassim, J. R., Collins, J. A., and Hilb, A. 1964. Metabolic studies in patients with hypercalciuria. *Clin. Sci.* **27:**463–482.
10. Murphy, G. P., and Schirmer, H. K. 1961. Nephrocalcinosis, urolithiasis and renal insufficiency in sarcoidosis. *J. Urol.* **86:**702–706.
11. Forbes, A. P., and Dempsey, E. 1963. *Nephrolithiasis Diseases of the Kidney.* M. B. Strauss and L. G. Welt, Eds. Little, Brown, Boston, pp. 714–727.
12. Kaplan, R. A., Snyder, W. H., Stewart, A., and Pak, C. Y. C. 1976. Metabolic effects of parathyroidectomy in asymptomatic primary hyperparathyroidism. *J. Clin. Endocrinol. Metab.* **42:**415–426.
13. Howard, J. E., Thomas, W. C., Jr., Mukai, T., Johnston, R. A., Jr., and Pascoe, B. J. 1962. The calcification of cartilage by urine, and a suggestion for therapy in patients with certain kinds of calculi. *Trans. Assoc. Am. Physicians* **75:**301–305.

14. Smith, L. H., Meyer, J. L., and McCall, J. T. 1973. Chemical nature of crystal inhibitors isolated from human urine. In *Urinary Calculi: Proceedings of the International Symposium on Renal Stone Research, Madrid, 1972.* L. Cifuentes Delatte, A. Rapado, and A. Hodgkinson, Eds. S. Karger, Basel and New York, pp. 318–327.

15. Takasaki, E. 1972. The magnesium:calcium ratio in the concentrated urines of patients with calcium oxalate calculi. *Invest. Urol.* **10**:147–150.

16. McIntosh, H. W., and Seraglia, M. 1963. Urinary excretion of calcium and citrate in normal individuals and stone formers with variation in calcium intake. *Can. Med. Assoc. J.* **89**:1242–1243.

17. Revusova, V., Zvara, V., and Gratzlova, J. 1973. Urinary zinc excretion in patients with urolithiasis. *Urol. Int.* **28**:72–79.

18. Robertson, W. G., Knowles, F., and Peacock, M. 1976. Urinary acid mucopolysaccharide inhibitors of calcium oxalate crystallization. In *Urolithiasis Research.* H. Fleisch, W. G. Robertson, L. H. Smith, and W. Vahlensieck, Eds. Plenum Press, New York, pp. 331–334.

19. Fleisch, H. 1977. Personal communication.

20. Finlayson, B., and Roth, R. 1973. Appraisal of calcium oxalate solubility in sodium chloride and sodium–calcium chloride solutions. *Urology* **1**:142–144.

21. Williams, H. E., 1976. Oxalic acid: Absorption, excretion and metabolism. In *Urolithiasis Research.* H. Fleisch, W. G. Robertson, L. H. Smith, and W. Vahlensieck, Eds. Plenum Press, New York, pp. 181–188.

22. Earnest, D. L., Williams, H. E., and Admirand, W. H. 1975. A physicochemical basis for treatment of enteric hyperoxaluria. *Trans. Assoc. Am. Physicians.* **88**:224–234.

23. Pak, C. Y. C., East, C., Sanzenbacher, L. J., Delea, C. S., and Bartter, F. C. 1972. Gastrointestinal calcium absorption in nephrolithiasis. *J. Clin. Endocrinol. Metab.* **35**:261–270.

24. Pak, C. Y. C. 1976. Idiopathic renal lithiasis: New developments in evaluation and treatment. In *Urolithiasis Research.* H. Fleisch, W. G. Robertson, L. H. Smith, and W. Vahlensieck, Eds. Plenum Press, New York, pp. 213–224.

25. Nordin, B. E. C., Peacock, M., and Wilkinson, R. 1972. Hypercalciuria and calcium stone disease. In *Clinics in Endocrinol. and Metabolism.* I. McIntyre, Ed. W. B. Saunders, Philadelphia, pp. 169–183.

26. Coe, F. L., Canterbury, J. M., Firpo, J. J., and Reiss, E. 1973. Evidence for secondary hyperparathyroidism in idiopathic hypercalciuria. *J. Clin. Invest.* **52**:134–142.

27. Agus, Z. S., Gardner, L. B., Beck, L. H., and Goldberg, M. 1973. Effects of parathyroid hormone on renal tubular reabsorption of calcium, sodium, and phosphate. *Am. J. Physiol.* **224**:1143–1148.

28. Pak, C. Y. C., Kaplan, R. A., Bone, H., Townsend, J., and Waters, O. 1975. A simple test for the diagnosis of absorptive, resorptive, and renal hypercalciurias. *N. Engl. J. Med.* **292**:497–500.

29. Barilla, D., Tolentino, R., Kaplan, R. A., and Pak, C. Y. C. Selective effect of thiazide on the intestinal absorption of calcium in absorptive and renal hypercalciurias. *Metabolism*. In press.
30. Henneman, P. H., Benedict, P. H., Forbes, A. P., and Dudley, H. R. 1958. Idiopathic hypercalciuria. *N. Engl. J. Med.* **259**:802–807.
31. Nordin, B. E. C., Peacock, M., and Marshall, D. H. 1976. Calcium excretion and hypercalciuria. In *Urolithiasis Research*. H. Fleisch, W. G. Robertson, L. H. Smith, and W. Vahlensieck, Eds. Plenum Press, New York, pp. 101–115.
32. Shen, F., Baylink, D., Nielson, R., Hughes, M., and Haussler, M. 1975. Increased serum 1,25-dihydroxycholecalciferol (1,25-diOHD₃) in patients with idiopathic hypercalciuria (IH). *Clin. Res.* **23A**:423.
33. Lemann, J., Gray, R. W., and Dominguez, J. H. 1976. 25-OH-vitamin D metabolism in calcium stone formers. In *Urolithiasis Research*. H. Fleisch, W. G. Robertson, L. H. Smith, and W. Vahlensieck, Eds. Plenum Press, New York, pp. 467–472.
34. Albright, F., Henneman, P., Benedict, P. H., and Forbes, A. P., 1953. Idiopathic hypercalciuria. *J. Clin. Endocrinol. Metab.* **13**:860.
35. Liberman, U. A., Sperling, O., Atsmon, A., Frank, M., Modan, M., and deVries, A. 1968. Metabolic and calcium kinetics studies in idiopathic hypercalciuria. *J. Clin. Invest.* **47**:2580–2590.
36. Edwards, N. A., and Hodgkinson, A. 1965. Metabolic studies in patients with idiopathic hypercalciuria. *Clin. Sci.* **29**:143–157.
37. Peacock, M., Hodgkinson, A., and Nordin, B. E. C. 1967. Importance of dietary calcium in the definition of hypercalciuria. *Br. Med. J.* **3**:469–471.
38. Dent, C. E., Harper, M., and Parfitt, A. M. 1964. The effect of cellulose phosphate on calcium metabolism in patients with hypercalciuria. *Clin. Sci.* **27**:417–425.
39. Peacock, M., and Nordin, B. E. C. 1968. Tubular reabsorption of calcium in normal and hypercalciuric subjects. *J. Clin. Pathol.* **21**:353–358.
40. Finn, W. F., Cerilli, G. J., and Ferris, T. F. 1970. Transplantation of a kidney from a patient with idiopathic hypercalciuria. *N. Engl. J. Med.* **283**:1450–1451.
41. Pronove, P., Bell, N. H., and Bartter, F. C. 1961. Production of hypercalciuria by phosphorus deprivation on a low calcium intake: A new clinical test for hyperparathyroidism. *Metabolism* **10**:364–371.
42. Pak, C. Y. C. 1972. Effects of cellulose phosphate and of sodium phosphate on the formation product and activity product of brushite in urine. *Metabolism* **21**:447–453.
43. Wills, M. R., Gill, J. R., Jr., and Bartter, F. C. 1969. The interrelationships of calcium and sodium excretions. *Clin. Sci. (Oxford)* **37**:621–630.
44. McCance, R. A., Widdowson, E. M., and Lehmann, H. 1942. The effect of protein intake on the absorption of calcium and magnesium. *Biochem. J.* **36**:686–691.

45. Murad, F., and Pak, C. Y. C. 1972. Urinary excretion of adenosine 3′,5′-monophosphate and guanosine 3′,5′-monophosphate. *N. Engl. J. Med.* **286:**1382–1387.

46. Shaw, J. W., Oldham, S. B., Rosoff, L., Bethune, J. E., and Fichman, M. P. 1977. Urinary cyclic AMP analyzed as a function of the serum calcium and parathyroid hormone in the differential diagnosis of hypercalcemia. *J. Clin. Invest.* **59:**14–21.

47. Arnaud, C. D., Hang, S. T., and Littledike, T. 1971. Radioimmunoassay of human parathyroid hormone in serum. *J. Clin. Invest.* **50:**21–34.

48. Reiss, E., and Canterbury, J. M. 1969. Primary hyperparathyroidism. Application of radioimmunoassay to differentiation of adenoma and hyperplasia and to preoperative localization of hyperfunctioning parathyroid glands. *N. Engl. J. Med.* **280:**1381–1385.

49. Bell, N. H., Gill, J. R., Jr., and Bartter, F. C. 1964. On the abnormal calcium absorption in sarcoidosis. *Am. J. Med.* **36:**500–513.

50. Lemann, J., Jr., Litzow, J. R., and Lennon, E. J. 1967. Studies of the mechanism by which chronic metabolic acidosis augments urinary calcium excretion in man. *J. Clin. Invest.* **46:**1318–1328.

51. Kaplan, R. A., Haussler, M. R., Deftos, L. J., Bone, H., and Pak, C. Y. C. The role of 1α,25-dihydroxycholecalciferol in the mediation of intestinal hyperabsorption of calcium in primary hyperparathyroidism and absorptive hypercalciuria. *J. Clin. Invest.* **59:**756–760.

52. McGeown, M. D. 1960. Heredity in renal stone disease. *Clin. Sci.* **19:**465–471.

53. Resnick, M., Pridgen, D. B., and Goodman, H. O. 1968. Genetic disposition to formation of calcium oxalate renal calculi. *N. Engl. J. Med.* **278:**1313–1318.

54. Haussler, M. R., Bursac, K. M., Bone, H., and Pak, C. Y. C. 1975. Increased circulating 1α,25-dihydroxyvitamin D_3 in patients with primary hyperparathyroidism. *Clin. Res.* **23:**322A.

55. Garabedian, M., Holick, M. F., DeLuca, H. F., and Boyle, I. T. 1973. Control of 25-hydroxycholecalciferol metabolism by parathyroid glands. *Proc. Natl. Acad. Sci. U.S.A.* **69:**1673–1676.

56. Hughes, M. R., Brumbaugh, P. F., Haussler, M. R., Wergedal, J. E., and Baylink, D. J. 1975. Regulation of serum 1α,25-dihydroxyvitamin D by calcium and phosphate in the rat. *Science* **190:**578–580.

57. Pak, C. Y. C. 1973. Sodium cellulose phosphate: Mechanism of action and effect on mineral metabolism. *J. Clin. Pharmacol.* **13:**15–27.

58. Hayashi, Y., Kaplan, R. A., and Pak, C. Y. C. 1975. Effect of sodium cellulose phosphate therapy on crystallization of calcium oxalate in urine. *Metabolism* **24:**1273–1278.

59. Marshall, R. W., and Barry, H. 1972. Urine saturation and the formation of calcium-containing renal calculi: The effects of various forms of therapy. In *Urinary Calculi: Proceedings of the International Symposium on Renal Stone*

Research, Madrid, 1972. L. Cifuentes Delatte, A. Rapado, and A. Hodgkinson, Eds. Karger, Basel and New York, pp. 164–169.

60. Rapado, A., Delatte, L. C., Villarino, J. A., and Sanchez-Martin, J. A. 1970. Treatment of idiopathic hypercalciuria with sodium cellulose phosphate. *Rev. Clin. Esp*. **119**:61–66.
61. Rose, A. G., and Harrison, A. R. 1974. The incidence, investigation, and treatment of idiopathic hypercalciuria. *Br. J. Urol*. **46**:261–274.
62. Blacklock, N. J., and MacLeod, M. A. 1974. The effect of cellulose phosphate on intestinal absorption and urinary excretion of calcium. *Br. J. Urol*. **46**:385–392.
63. Pak, C. Y. C., Delea, C. S., and Bartter, F. C. 1974. Successful treatment of recurrent nephrolithiasis (calcium stones) with cellulose phosphate. *N. Engl. J. Med*. **290**:175–180.
64. Pak, C. Y. C., Wortsman, J., Bennett, J. E., Delea, C. S., and Bartter, F. C. 1968. Control of hypercalcemia with cellulose phosphate. *J. Clin. Endocrinol. Metab*. **28**:1829–1832.
65. Yendt, E. R., Guay, G. F., and Garcia, D. A. 1970. The use of thiazides in the prevention of renal calculi. *Can. Med. Assoc. J*. **102**:614–620.
66. Lamberg, B. A., and Kuhlback, B. 1959. Effect of chlorothiazide and hydrochlorothiazide on the excretion of calcium in the urine. *Scand. J. Clin. Lab. Invest*. **11**:351–357.
67. Middler, S., Pak, C. Y. C., Murad, F., and Bartter, F. C. 1973. Thiazide diuretics and calcium metabolism. *Metabolism* **22**:139–146.
68. Brickman, A. S., Massry, S. G., and Coburn, J. W. 1972. Changes in serum and urinary calcium during treatment with hydrochlorothiazide: Studies on mechanisms. *J. Clin. Invest*. **51**:945–954.
69. Pak, C. Y. C. 1973. Hydrochlorothiazide therapy in nephrolithiasis: Effect on urinary activity product and formation product of brushite. *Clin. Pharmacol. Ther*. **14**:209–217.
70. Pak, C. Y. C., Ruskin, B., and Diller, E. 1972. Enhancement of renal excretion of zinc by hydrochlorothiazide. *Clin. Chim. Acta* **39**:511–517.
71. Cohanim, M., and Yendt, E. R. 1975. The effects of thiazides on serum and urinary zinc in patients with renal calculi. *Johns Hopkins Med. J*. **136**:137–141.
72. Pickelman, J., Payloyan, F., Forland, M., and Strauss, F. H. 1968. Thiazide induced parathyroid stimulation. *Clin. Res*. **16**:468.
73. Costanzo, L. S., Moses, A. M., Janardhana Rao, K., and Weiner, I. M. 1975. Dissociation of calcium and sodium clearances in patients with hypoparathyroidism by infusion of chlorothiazide. *Metabolism* **24**:1367–1373.
74. Costanzo, L. S., and Weiner, I. M. 1974. On the hypocalciuric action of chlorothiazide. *J. Clin. Invest*. **54**:628–637.
75. Woelfel, A., Kaplan, R. A., and Pak, C. Y. C. 1977. Effect of hydrochlorothiazide therapy on the crystallization of calcium oxalate in urine. *Metabolism* **26**:201–205.

76. Gursel, E. 1970. Effects of diuretics on renal and intestinal handling of calcium. *N. Y. State J. Med.* **70:**399–405.

77. Duarte, C. G., Winnacker, J. L., Becker, K. L., and Pace, A. 1971. Thiazide-induced hypercalcemia. *N. Engl. J. Med.* **284:**828–830.

78. Parfitt, A. M. 1969. Chlorothiazide-induced hypercalcemia in juvenile osteoporosis and hyperparathyroidism. *N. Engl. J. Med.* **281:**55–59.

79. Banks, P. A. 1971. Acute pancreatitis. *Gastroenterology* **61:**382–397.

80. Forland, M., Strandjord, N. M., Paloyan, E., and Cox, A. 1968. Bone density studies in primary hyperparathyroidism. *Arch. Intern. Med.* **122:**236–240.

81. Fleisch, H., Bisaz, S., and Care, A. D. 1964. Effect of orthophosphate on urinary pyrophosphate excretion and the prevention of urolithiasis. *Lancet* **1:**1065–1067.

82. Reiss, E., Canterbury, J. M., Bercovitz, M. A., and Kaplan, E. L. 1970. The role of phosphate in the secretion of parathyroid hormone in man. *J. Clin. Invest.* **40:**2146–2149.

83. Smith, L. H., Thomas, W. C., Jr., and Arnaud, C. D. 1972. Orthophosphate therapy in calcium renal lithiasis. In *Urinary Calculi: Proceedings of the International Symposium on Renal Stone Research, Madrid, 1972.* L. Cifuentes Delatte, A. Rapado, and A. Hodgkinson, Eds. Karger, Basel and New York, pp. 188–197.

84. Raisz, L. G., and Niemann, I. 1969. Effect of phosphate, calcium and magnesium on bone resorption and hormonal responses in tissue culture. *Endocrinology* **85:**446–452.

85. Spaulding, S. W., and Walser, M. 1970. Treatment of experimental hypercalcemia with oral phosphate. *J. Clin. Endocrinol.* **31:**531–538.

86. Dudley, F. J., and Blackburn, C. R. B. 1970. Extraskeletal calcification complicating oral neutral-phosphate therapy. *Lancet* **2:**628–630.

87. Pak, C. Y. C. 1977. Idiopathic hypercalciuria. In *Advances in Experimental Medicine and Biology, Vol. 81: Phosphate Metabolism.* S. G. Massry and E. Ritz, Eds. Plenum, New York, pp. 309–317.

88. Bernstein, D. S., and Newton, R. 1966. The effect of oral sodium phosphate on the formation of renal calculi and on idiopathic hypercalciuria. *Lancet* **2:**1105–1107.

89. Ettinger, B., and Kolb, F. 1973. Inorganic phosphate treatment of nephrolithiasis. *Am. J. Med.* **55:**32–37.

90. Ettinger, B. 1976. Recurrent nephrolithiasis: Natural history and effect of phosphate therapy. A double-blind control study. *Am. J. Med.* **61:**200–206.

91. Jowsey, J., Reiss, E., and Canterbury, J. M. 1974. Long-term effects of high phosphate intake on parathyroid hormone levels and bone metabolism. *Acta Orthop. Scand.* **45:**801–808.

92. Goldsmith, R. S., Jowsey, J., Dube, W. J., Riggs, B. L., Arnaud, C. D., and Kelly, P. J. 1976. Effects of phosphorus supplementation on serum

parathyroid hormone and bone morphology in osteoporosis. *J. Clin. Endocrinol. Metab.* **43:**523–532.

93. Francis, M. D. 1969. The inhibition of calcium hydroxyapatite crystal growth by polyphosphonates and polyphosphates. *Calcif. Tissue Res.* **3:**151–162.

94. Michael, W. R., King, W. R., and Wakim, J. M. 1972. Metabolism of disodium ethane-1-hydroxy-1,1-diphosphonate (disodium etidronate) in the rat, rabbit, dog and monkey. *Toxicol. Applied Pharmacol.* **21:**503–515.

95. Ohata, M., and Pak, C. Y. C. 1974. Preliminary study of the treatment of nephrolithiasis (calcium stones) with diphosphonate. *Metabolism* **23:**1167–1173.

96. Recker, R. R., Hassing, G. S., Lau, J. R., and Saville, P. D. 1973. The hyperphosphatemic effect of disodium ethane-1-hydroxy-1, 1-diphosphonate (EHDP®): Renal handling of phosphorus and the renal response to parathyroid hormone. *J. Lab. Clin. Med.* **81:**258–266.

97. Kaplan R. A., Geho, W. B., Poindexter, C., Haussler, M., Dietz, G. W., and Pak, C. Y. C. Metabolic effects of diphosphonate in primary hyperparathyroidism. *J. Clin. Pharmacol.* **17:**410–419.

98. Hill, L. F., Lumb, G. A., Mawer, E. B., and Stanbury, S. W. 1973. Indirect inhibition of the biosynthesis of 1,25-dihydroxycholecalciferol in rats treated with a diphosphonate. *Clin. Sci.* **44:**335–347.

99. Ohata, M., and Pak, C. Y. C. 1973. The effect of diphosphonate on calcium phosphate crystallization in urine *in vitro. Kidney Int.* **4:**401–406.

100. Fraser, D., Russell, R. G. G., Pohler, O., Robertson, W. G., and Fleisch, H. 1972. The influence of disodium ethane-1-hydroxy-1,1-diphosphonate (EHDP) on the development of experimentally induced urinary stones in rats. *Clin. Sci.* **42:**197–207.

101. Pak, C. Y. C., Ohata, M., and Holt, K. 1975. Effect of diphosphonate on crystallization of calcium oxalate *in vitro. Kidney Int.* **7:**154–160.

102. Robertson, W. G., Peacock, M., Marshall, R. W., and Knowles, F. 1974. The effect of ethane-1-hydroxy-1,1-diphosphonate (EHDP) on calcium oxalate crystalluria in recurrent renal stone-formers. *Clin. Sci. Mol. Med.* **27:**13–22.

103. Pak, C. Y. C. 1977. Physicochemical and clinical aspects of nephrolithiasis. *Proceedings of an International Colloquium on Renal Lithiasis.* B. Finlayson and W. C. Thomas, Jr., Eds. University of Florida Press, Gainesville, pp. 257–275.

104. Francis, M. D., Russell, R. G. G., and Fleisch, H. 1969. Diphosphonates inhibit formation of calcium phosphate crystals *in vitro* and pathological calcification *in vivo. Science* **165:**1264–1266.

105. Bone, H., Britton, F., and Pak, C. Y. C. In preparation.

106. Jowsey, J., Holley, K. E., and Lemann, J. W. 1970. Effect of sodium etidronate on adult cats. *J. Lab. Clin. Med.* **76:**126–133.

107. Sutor, D. J. 1969. Growth studies of calcium oxalate in the presence of various ions and compounds. *Br. J. Urol.* **41**:171–178.
108. Meyer, J. L., and Smith, L. H. 1975. Growth of calcium oxalate crystals. II. Inhibition by natural urinary crystal growth inhibitors. *Invest. Urol.* **13**:36–39.
109. Fetner, C., Barilla, D. E., and Pak, C. Y. C. In preparation.
110. Barilla, D. E., Notz, C., Kennedy, D., and Pak, C. Y. C. Renal oxalate excretion following oral oxalate loads in patients with ileal disease and with renal and absorptive hypercalciurias: Effect of calcium and magnesium. *Am. J. Med.* In press.
111. Hammersten, G. 1956. *Etiologic Factor in Renal Lithiasis*. A. J. Pruitt, Ed. Charles C. Thomas, Springfield, Illinois, pp. 96.
112. Dobbins, J. W., and Binder, H. J. 1977. Importance of the colon in enteric hyperoxaluria. *N. Engl. J. Med.* **296**:298–301.
113. Clark, I. 1969. Effects of magnesium on calcium and phosphate metabolism in parathyroidectomized rats. *Endocrinology* **85**:1103–1113.
114. Pak, C. Y. C., and Diller, E. C. 1969. Ionic interaction with bone mineral. V. Effect of Mg^{2+}, $citrate^{3-}$, F^-, and $SO_4{}^{2-}$ on the solubility, dissolution and growth of bone mineral. *Calcif. Tissue Res.* **4**:69–77.
115. Chase, L. R., and Slatopolsky, E. 1974. Secretion and metabolic efficacy of parathyroid hormone in patients with severe hypomagnesemia. *J. Clin. Endocrinol. Metab.* **38**:363–371.
116. Pak, C. Y. C. 1973. Calcareous renal stones. *Medcom Famous Teaching in Medicine*. Medcom, New York, pp. 1–35.
117. Murphy, F. J., Zelman, S., and Mau, W. 1965. Ascorbic acid as a urinary acidifying agent. 2. Its adjunctive role in chronic urinary infection. *J. Urol.* **94**:300–303.
118. Murphy, F. J., and Zelman, S. 1965. Ascorbic acid as a urinary acidifying agent. 1. Comparison with the ketogenic effect of fasting. *J. Urol.* **94**:297–299.
119. McDonald, D. F., and Murphy, G. P. 1959. Bacteriostatic and acidifying effects of methionine, hydrolyzed casein and ascorbic acid on the urine. *N. Engl. J. Med.* **261**:803–805.
120. Pauling, L. 1970. *Vitamin C and the Common Cold*. W. H. Freeman and Co., San Francisco.
121. Coulehan, J. L., Reisinger, K. S., Rogers, K. D., and Bradley, D. W. 1974. Vitamin C prophylaxis in a boarding school. *N. Engl. J. Med.* **290**:6–10.
122. Karlowski, T. R., Chalmers, T. C., Frenkel, L. D., Kapikian, A. Z., Lewis, T. L., and Lynch, J. M. 1975. Ascorbic acid for the common cold: A prophylactic and therapeutic trial. *J. Am. Med. Assoc.* **231**: 1038–1042.
123. Coulehan, J. L., Eberhard, S., Kapner, L., Taylor, F., Rogers, K., and Garry, P. 1976. Vitamin C and acute illness in Navajo school children. *N. Engl. J. Med.* **295**:973–977.

124. Lamden, M. P., and Chrystowski, G. A. 1954. Urinary oxalate excretion by man following ascorbic acid ingestion. *Proc. Soc. Exp. Biol. Med.* **85:**190–192.
125. Takenouchi, K., Aso, K., Kawase, K., Ichikawa, H., and Shiomi, T. 1966. On the metabolites of ascorbic acid, especially oxalic acid, eliminated in urine, following the administration of large amounts of ascorbic acid. *J. Vitaminol.* **12:**49–58.
126. Takiguchi, H., Furuyama, S., and Shimazono, N. 1966. Urinary oxalic acid excretion by man following ingestion of large amounts of ascorbic acid. *J. Vitaminol.* **12:**307–312.
127. Briggs, M. H., Garcia-Webb, P., and Davies, P. 1973. Urinary oxalate and vitamin-C supplements. *Lancet* **2:**201.
128. Pak, C. Y. C. 1972. Nephrolithiasis (Ca-containing). *Acta Endocrinol. Panam.* **3:**45–52.

Chapter 4

Primary Hyperparathyroidism and Other Causes of Hypercalcemia

Primary hyperparathyroidism continues to be one of the leading causes of Ca urolithiasis.[1-5] Although the exact pathogenetic mechanism for the stone formation in primary hyperparathyroidism has not been clarified, effective control of urolithiasis can usually be achieved by the surgical removal of abnormal parathyroid tissue.[6,7] This condition is not too difficult to diagnose when it is fully manifested. However, primary hyperparathyroidism may escape detection in its subtle presentation and may be confused with other forms of Ca urolithiasis.[8,9] This difficulty has resulted in the recommendation of parathyroid exploration, albeit infrequently, in renal[10] and absorptive[11] hypercalciurias. The following cases illustrate examples of such useless surgery.

Case 1. A 39-year-old woman was initially referred for evaluation of Ca urolithiasis. She had allegedly passed more than 300 stones spontaneously during the preceding 14 years. Stone analysis had disclosed the presence of both apatite (Ca phosphate) and Ca oxalate. No surgery for the removal of stone had been required. She had numerous hospital admissions and emergency visits for renal colic, for which she received Demerol. Her emotional stability and compliance with the treatment program were questioned by the referring physician.

The evaluation disclosed normal serum Ca of 9.5 mg% and P of 3.6 mg%. She had hypercalciuria of 260–288 mg/day on a diet of 400 mg Ca/day. Moreover, she had a high fasting urinary Ca of 0.16 mg/mg creatinine, a finding indicating that she had an impaired renal tubular reabsorption of Ca or an excessive skeletal mobilization of Ca.[12,13] The renal excretion of cyclic AMP (cAMP) and serum immunoreactive parathyroid hormone (iPTH) were elevated. It was therefore felt that she probably suffered from renal hypercalciuria with secondary hyperparathyroidism.[10,13] The abdominal roentgenogram disclosed the presence of bilateral radiopaque renal calculi.

Unfortunately, she failed to adhere to the recommended medical therapy, and was eventually lost to follow-up. One year later, she was evaluated elsewhere for recurrent nephrolithiasis. She was considered to suffer from normocalcemic primary hyperparathyroidism[7,8,14−16] because of high circulating concentration of PTH and hypercalciuria. During parathyroid exploration, all glands were reportedly slightly enlarged. Two glands were resected; the remaining glands were biopsied. Parathyroid hyperplasia was found in all glands.

The parathyroidectomy did not correct the hypercalciuria or abate stone formation. Evaluation disclosed that she was still suffering from renal hypercalciuria. Serum Ca was 9.2 mg% and P 3.1 mg%. She had hypercalciuria of 389 mg/day and a high fasting urinary Ca of 0.22 mg/mg creatinine.[13] Serum iPTH and urinary AMP were both elevated.

Case 2. This 57-year-old plumber passed his first renal stone when he was 22 years old. He was well until 30 years of age, when he began to pass numerous renal stones of Ca oxalate and Ca phosphate at a frequency of nearly two per month. While most of the stones were passed spontaneously, some had to be removed surgically because of obstruction. Six nephrolithotomies were required, three from each kidney. He found his situation disdainful. As a stoic, he could tolerate renal colic, but he found himself at a psychological disadvantage. "Some fix for a plumber to be in, not being able to p---," he complained.

At 50 years of age, an evaluation elsewhere disclosed a serum Ca concentration of 10.0 mg%, P of 3.0 mg%, and alkaline phosphatase of 10 King–Armstrong units. Urinary Ca was high at 350 mg/day. He was considered to have an abnormal parathyroid function, on the basis of high renal P clearance and reduced renal tubular reabsorption of P. During parathyroid exploration, four normal glands were found.

The parathyroid surgery did not affect recurrent renal stone formation. At 53 years of age, a more extensive evaluation disclosed that he suffered from absorptive hypercalciuria.[11-13]

The cases described above emphasize the importance of an accurate diagnosis of primary hyperparathyroidism before parathyroid surgery is undertaken. The following is a review of current trends in the clinical presentations, pathogenesis, diagnostic criteria, and indications for parathyroidectomy in primary hyperparathyroidism. Because hypercalcemia is an important concomitant of primary hyperparathyroidism, a definition of hypercalcemia is in order.

DEFINITION OF HYPERCALCEMIA

A clear understanding of the physicochemical state of calcium in blood and of calcium homeostatic control is required before hypercalcemia may be properly defined.

State of Calcium in Plasma

The total serum Ca (Ca_T) is the sum of free ionized Ca (Ca^{2+}) and complexed Ca (CaX).

$$Ca_T = Ca^{2+} + CaX$$

The complexed Ca is composed of diffusible and nondiffusible components.[17] The diffusible component, comprising approximately one eighth of Ca_T, represents formation of soluble complexes, principally with phosphate, sulfate, citrate, and bicarbonate. The nondiffusible component, accounting for about one third of Ca_T, reflects binding to proteins, principally albumin. Important factors that affect the complexation of Ca are the pH and concentration of ligands, particularly of albumin and phosphate. Reduction in pH inhibits complexation of albumin, and alters the amount of $CaHPO_4$ and $CaH_2PO_4^+$ complexes by affecting the dissociation of phosphate.[18-20]

The critically important fraction in pathophysiology is Ca^{2+}. Unfortunately, few reliable techniques are available for its direct analysis. Two approaches allow indirect measurement of Ca^{2+}. The diffusible component, comprising approximately 75% of Ca_T, can be obtained by ultrafiltration.[21,22] The Ca^{2+} can then be determined by "subtracting" soluble complexes of Ca (obtained by means of a computer program) from ultrafiltrable Ca.[18-20] Alternatively, the calcium ion activity (α_{Ca}^{2+}) can be determined with the Ca ion electrode[23,24]:

$$\alpha_{Ca^{2+}} = \gamma_{Ca^{2+}} \cdot C_{Ca^{2+}}$$

Since the ionic strength of serum approximates 0.15, the activity coefficient of Ca (γ) can be assumed to be constant[25] at approximately 0.35. The standard curve can be drawn from values of $\alpha_{Ca^{2+}}$ (electrode potential) at various Ca^{2+} concentrations in artificial solutions of constant ionic strength (of 0.15).[24] The concentration of Ca^{2+} ($C_{Ca^{2+}}$) can be obtained by interpolation from the standard curve.

When neither of the methods described above is available, Ca^{2+} can be estimated as follows: Using the nomogram of Moore,[23] calculate protein-bound Ca from serum pH and albumin concentration. Assume the amount of soluble Ca complexes to be 0.3 mM.[17] Subtract protein-bound Ca and soluble Ca complexes from Ca_T to obtain Ca^{2+}.

Calcium Homeostatic Mechanisms

Under normal circumstances, the circulating concentration of Ca^{2+} is maintained within a narrow range by various homeostatic mechanisms. Three types of homeostatic control mechanisms are probably involved in the maintenance of plasma Ca concentration: one hormonal, another physicochemical, and the third physiological.

Hormonal Regulation. Parathyroid hormone (PTH) is recognized as one of the most important factors in Ca homeostasis. The secretion of this hormone is carefully regulated by the plasma concentration of Ca^{2+}.[26] When plasma Ca^{2+} is depressed, the secretion of PTH is stimulated. The stimulation of PTH restores plasma Ca^{2+} to normal by increasing some or all of bone resorption,[27] intestinal Ca absorption,[28] and renal tubular reabsorption of Ca.[29] Conversely, when plasma Ca^{2+} is increased, the secretion of PTH is suppressed; plasma Ca^{2+} is thereby reduced toward normal.

Two other factors—1α,25-dihydroxycholecalciferol [1α,25-$(OH)_2D$] and calcitonin, have been implicated in Ca homeostasis. These hormones are each capable of altering plasma Ca^{2+} concentration; their secretion may be modified by the circulating concentration of Ca^{2+}.

Cholecalciferol, the native vitamin D formed in the skin on UV exposure, is biologically inactive.[30] It is hydroxylated in the liver to form 25-hydroxycholecalciferol, and is further converted in the kidney to 1α,25-$(OH)_2D$. Classic effects of 25-hydroxycholecalciferol and 1α,25-$(OH)_2D$ are the stimulation of intestinal Ca absorption[31] and promotion of bone resorption.[32] 1α,25-$(OH)_2D$ is more potent than the hepatic metabolite in these respects. Both metabolites augment the renal tubular reabsorption of Ca.[33] The net effect of these actions is an increase in the circulating concentration of Ca.

As with PTH, the secretion of 1α,25-$(OH)_2D$ is stimulated by low plasma Ca^{2+} and suppressed by high plasma Ca^{2+}.[30] The importance of 1α,25-$(OH)_2D$ in Ca homeostasis appears irrefutable. The synthesis and function of 1α,25-$(OH)_2D$ appears to be closely related to the state of parathyroid function. Its secretion is stimulated in conditions of PTH excess.[34] This vitamin D metabolite may be an important mediator for the PTH-stimulated intestinal Ca absorption.[28] In primary hyperparathyroidism, for example, the increased absorption of Ca was positively correlated with the increased circulating levels of $1\alpha,25\text{-}(OH)_2D$[35] [See Figure 13 (Chapter 3)].

Calcitonin, a polypeptide hormone produced by parafollicular cells of the thyroid gland, lowers serum Ca concentration by inhibiting bone resorption[36] and augmenting renal excretion of Ca.[37] Its effect on intestinal Ca transport is controversial.[38] The secretion of calcitonin is also dependent on plasma concentration of Ca,[39] though opposite in direction to that of PTH and $1\alpha,25\text{-}(OH)_2D$. Thus, when plasma Ca^{2+} is increased, the enhanced secretion of calcitonin may serve to lower plasma Ca^{2+} toward normal. Unfortunately, the biological significance of calcitonin in health has been questioned. When the endogenous production of calcitonin is largely eliminated by thyroidectomy, there is no evidence that a major disturbance of Ca homeostasis ensues.

Physicochemical Regulation.[17] It has been hypothesized that plasma concentrations of Ca^{2+} and phosphate reflect the solubility of the bone mineral. This hypothesis assumes that circulating concentrations of Ca^{2+} and phosphate are maintained at a constant product, representing saturation with respect to a particular phase of Ca phosphate in bone. This scheme could explain the decline in plasma Ca^{2+} that ensues from the rise in plasma phosphate. The circulating concentration of Ca^{2+} is expected to be maintained in a narrow range, insofar as the plasma concentration of phosphate does not fluctuate widely.

Unfortunately, various physicochemical studies have failed to identify the particular phase of Ca phosphate with which plasma Ca^{2+} and phosphate might be in steady state. They have shown the extracellular fluid to be supersaturated with respect to hydroxyapatite, the predominant mineral phase in bone, and undersaturated with respect to brushite $(CaHPO_4 \cdot 2H_2O)$,[17] the "precursor" phase of hydroxyapatite.[25,40,41] The results suggest that the interstitial fluid of bone, which is in steady state with bone mineral, is not equivalent to the extracellular fluid in ionic composition. It has therefore been postulated that a barrier or ion gradient exists between these two fluid compartments. The action of PTH, $1\alpha,25$-$(OH)_2D$, and calcitonin, for example, may be assumed to involve the regulation of this ionic gradient.

Physiological Regulation. The kidney may play an important role in Ca homeostasis by regulating the excretion of Ca.[42] This regulation is partly hormone-independent, since the renal excretion of Ca is a function of the filtered load of Ca. For example, the kidneys may remove as much as 800 mg Ca/day while maintaining plasma Ca in the normal range. It is also hormone-dependent, since renal tubular reabsorption may be modified by hormonal action, particularly by PTH. When serum Ca is raised, the renal excretion of Ca is promoted from the increased filtered load of Ca and reduced renal tubular reabsorption of Ca consequent to parathyroid suppression.[29] When serum Ca is reduced, as from malabsorption of Ca, the renal excretion of Ca may decrease from a fall in renal filtered load of Ca and an increase in renal tubular reabsorption of Ca associated with parathyroid stimulation.

Normal Serum Calcium Concentration

The normal range for serum Ca has become more refined consequent to the improved methods for the analysis of total Ca. Extensive studies by Keating *et al.*[43] indicate that serum level declines with age and is lower in normal women than in normal men. Their nomogram may be useful, provided there are no significant abnormalities in pH or in protein concentrations.

The most reliable means of defining normocalcemia, especially in states of disturbed acid–base balance or protein metabolism, is by the determination of plasma Ca^{2+}. If Ca ion electrode is not available, Ca^{2+} may be estimated from total Ca, making an adjustment for albumin concentration and pH.

Hypercalcemia: Loss of Calcium Homeostatic Control

Hypercalcemia may be viewed as the sequela of the loss of Ca homeostatic control. For it to develop, there must be, first, a sufficient, unabated "input" of Ca into the circulating fluid, as might occur from a continued excessive rate of bone resorption or of intestinal Ca absorption. Such a situation might result from the loss of hormonal regulation, as in primary hyperparathyroidism. Second, the extent of the input of Ca in the circulating fluid must exceed the capacity of the kidneys (and of the intestines) to remove the Ca load.

PRIMARY HYPERPARATHYROIDISM

In primary hyperparathyroidism, Ca homeostatic control is lost consequent to an excessive PTH secretion.[2] Thus, PTH is secreted by adenomatous or hyperplastic parathyroid tissue in amounts that are inappropriately high for the level of circulating Ca^{2+}. Hypercalcemia develops from the combined effects of PTH-induced stimulation of bone resorption,[32] intestinal Ca absorption,[28] and renal tubular reabsorption of Ca.[29] Hypercalciuria is often found. Even though PTH augments the renal tubular reabsorption of Ca, this action of the hormone is usually insufficient to overcome the increased renal filtered load of Ca associated with hypercalcemia.[11]

The major symptoms of primary hyperparathyroidism may be ascribed to the PTH-induced resorption of bone, hypercalciuria, or hypercalcemia.

Pathogenesis of Bone Disease in Primary Hyperparathyroidism

The bone disease in primary hyperparathyroidism may take several forms. There may be bone cysts (brown tumors) or subperiosteal resorption. The most frequent sites of subperiosteal resorption are the phalanges and distal clavicles. Usually, the subperiosteal involvement appears as fraying of margins. In severe forms, granular demineralization of the skull may occur. Finally, the bone disease may appear as osteoporosis with vertebral compression.[44] The severity or the type of bone disease probably depends to some extent on the degree of PTH secretion. Brown tumor, osteitis fibrosa cystica, or extensive subperiosteal resorption is usually associated with high circulating levels of PTH and large glandular size.[45] Osteoporosis, particularly in postmenopausal white women, may result from a mild to moderate stimulation of PTH for a prolonged period.[44]

There is ample evidence that PTH is required for the development of osteoporosis.[46,47] Osteoporosis is rarely encountered in hypoparathyroidism.[48] Osteoporosis of disuse[49] and low-Ca–

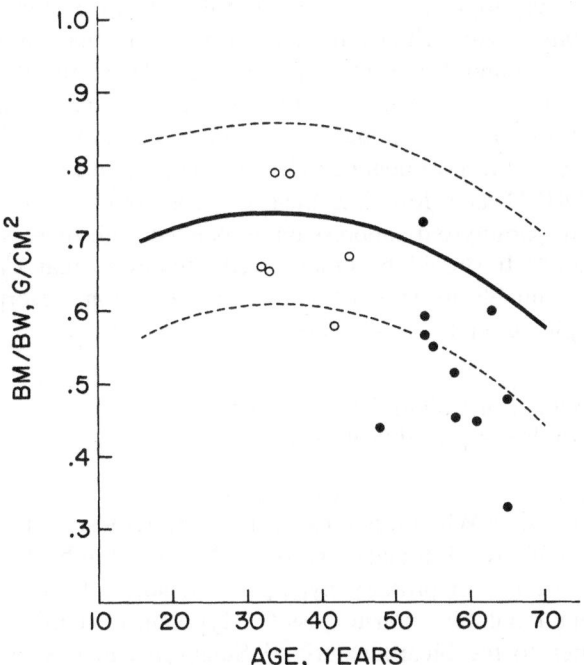

FIGURE 15. Bone density in white women patients with primary hyperparathyroidism. Solid and dashed curves indicate mean and 95% confidence limits on the observation for the control subjects. Each circle represents studies in a separate patient. (○) Values from premenopausal women; (●) values from postmenopausal women.

high-phosphate intake[50] do not develop in the absence of parathyroid glands. The metabolism of the bone cell in osteoporosis
resembles that in primary hyperparathyroidism.[51,52]

The association of osteoporosis with the postmenopausal state
emphasizes a potentially important relationship between estrogen
and PTH in the genesis of osteoporosis. Estrogen is believed to an-
tagonize the action of PTH on bone.[53,54] It has been shown to inhibit the PTH-induced resorption of bone *in vitro*.[53] It reduces
plasma concentration of Ca, as well as urinary Ca and hydroxy-
proline,[55,56] and may be useful in the treatment of postmenopausal
women with primary hyperparathyroidism.[56] Bone density by [125]I-
photon absorptiometry is reduced significantly in postmenopausal
white women with primary hyperparathyroidism than in age- and
sex-matched control subjects[57] (Figure 15). These results suggest
that loss of the "protective" action of estrogen against the PTH-
mediated bone resorption may contribute to the development of osteoporosis in the postmenopausal state. The reduced synthesis of
$1\alpha,25-(OH)_2D$ and low intestinal Ca absorption may be consequent to parathyroid suppression associated with increased bone
resorption.[58] It should be emphasized, however, that Caputo *et
al.*[59] were unable to demonstrate inhibition of bone resorption by
physiologic amounts of estrogens.

Pathogenesis of Calcium Urolithiasis in Primary Hyperparathyroidism

Nephrocalcinosis is much less commonly encountered than
nephrolithiasis.[3] When it is present, nephrocalcinosis is usually associated with renal tubular acidosis. The renal tubular acidosis
probably occurs in primary hyperparathyroidism from the PTH-
dependent renal bicarbonate loss.[60] Hypophosphatemia probably
contributes to the bicarbonaturia.[61] Staghorn calculus or struvite
stone may develop, especially if the condition is associated with
chronic urinary tract infection. The clinical presentation of nephrolithiasis in primary hyperparathyroidism may be indistinguishable
from that of absorptive hypercalciuria. However, predominantly

Ca phosphate stones may be more frequently encountered in primary hyperparathyroidism than in absorptive hypercalciuria.

Hypercalciuria is an important factor concerned with renal stone disease.[25,62,63] Hypercalciuria probably contributes to stone formation by rendering urine supersaturated with respect to brushite and Ca oxalate.[62] Urine samples from a majority of patients with primary hyperparathyroidism were supersaturated with respect to these Ca salts[62] [see Figures 4 and 5 (Chapter 2)]. The state of saturation was positively correlated with the urinary concentration of Ca. Virtually every patient with primary hyperparathyroidism and nephrolithiasis had hypercalciuria and urinary supersaturation with respect to brushite and Ca oxalate.

Hypercalciuria is not the sole factor, however, since certain patients with primary hyperparathyroidism do not form stones despite hypercalciuria and a supersaturated state of urine with respect to Ca salts. Recent studies suggest that there is in primary hyperparathyroidism an increased renal excretion of certain substances, which facilitate spontaneous precipitation of Ca phosphate and Ca oxalate. Thus, the formation product ratio (FPR) (limit of metastability) of brushite and Ca oxalate was lower in urine samples from many patients with primary hyperparathyroidism than in synthetic medium[62] (Figure 16). The result cannot be explained by a lack of inhibitor activity, since in the total absence of inhibitors, the FPR in urine should have approached that in synthetic medium and should not have fallen below it. The finding cited above is more compatible with the presence in urine of promoter(s) of nucleation.

Following parathyroidectomy, urine specimens became less saturated or undersaturated with respect to brushite[64] and Ca oxalate (Table V), commensurate with a fall in urinary Ca. Moreover, the FPR of Ca salts increased, a finding suggesting that the promoter activity, if it were present, had become less prominent. These studies indicate that the physicochemical basis for stone formation in primary hyperparathyroidism may be due at least in part to the supersaturated state and increased propensity for the precipitation of brushite and Ca oxalate in urine.

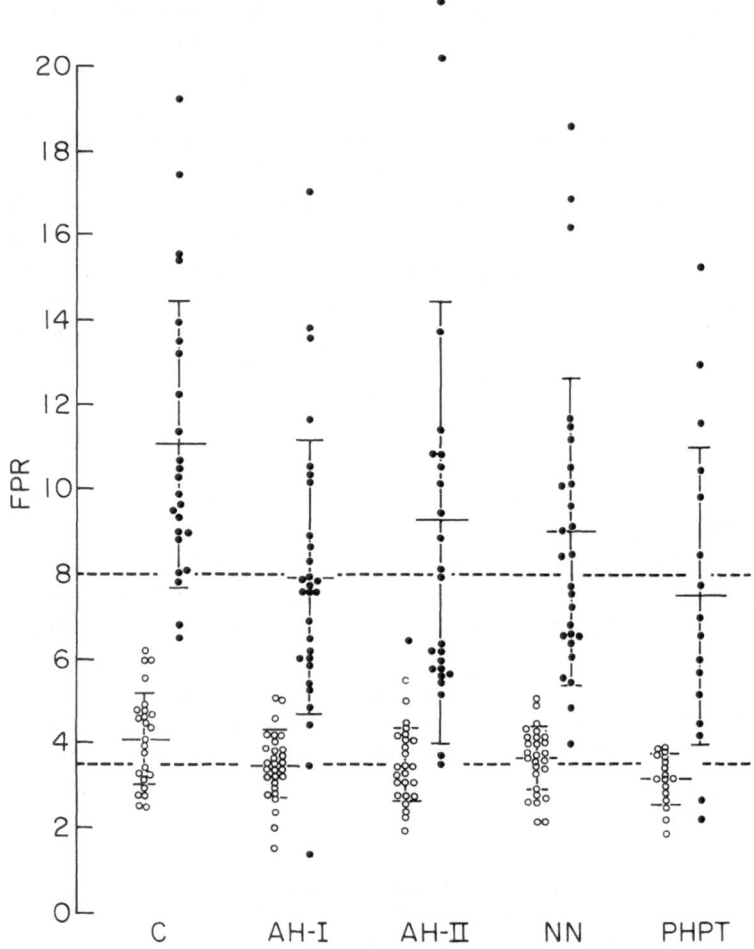

FIGURE 16. Formation product ratio (FPR) of brushite (○) and Ca oxalate (●). The upper horizontal dashed line indicates the FPR of Ca oxalate for a synthetic solution (devoid of inhibitors of nucleation). The lower horizontal dashed line represents the FPR of brushite for a synthetic solution. A value of 1 represents saturation; of greater than 1, supersaturation; and of less than 1, undersaturation. The horizontal bars represent means ± S.D. (C) Control group; (AH-I) absorptive hypercalciuria Type I; (AH-II) absorptive hypercalciuria Type II; (NN) normocalciuric nephrolithiasis; (PHPT) primary hyperparathyroidism.

TABLE V. Effect of Parathyroidectomy[a]

Ratio	Control	PTX
APR Ca oxalate	3.20 ± 1.48	1.53 ± 0.55[b]
FPR Ca oxalate	7.19 ± 3.16	12.99 ± 4.45[c]

[a]Effect of parathyroidectomy (PTX) on the urinary activity product ratio (APR) and the formation product ratio (FPR) of Ca oxalate in 7 patients with primary hyperparathyroidism. Results are presented as means ± S.D.
[b,c]$p < 0.05$[b] and $p < 0.001$[c] by paired Student's t test.

The nature of the promoter of nucleation is not known. Although monosodium urate may cause heterogeneous nucleation of Ca phosphate and Ca oxalate,[65-67] it is probably not the promoter sought in primary hyperparathyroidism. Even in undersaturated urine specimens in which the solid phase of monosodium urate cannot form, the promoter activity, as reflected by a reduced formation product ratio, was found. The promoter activity is not unique to the hyperparathyroid state, since it is probably also present in the urine of certain patients with absorptive hypercalciuria.[62] It is tempting to speculate that the promoter(s) may be analogous or similar to the organic matrix (or components of that matrix) found in stones, in intranephronic calculosis, or in microspherules (see Chapter 2). Once promoters have been identified, it is necessary to show that they are present in both primary hyperparathyroidism and absorptive hypercalciuria and that their renal excretion is reduced following parathyroidectomy.

The conclusion stated above does not exclude the participation of inhibitors of nucleation on stone formation in primary hyperparathyroidism. Thus, reduced renal excretion of inhibitors could facilitate spontaneous precipitation of Ca salts in urine by lowering the formation product ratio. However, no study has been performed to separate the effects of inhibitors from those of promoters. Moreover, the contention that the renal excretion of pyrophosphate is increased in primary hyperparathyroidism has been disputed.[68,69]

Pathogenesis of Other Symptoms of Primary Hyperparathyroidism

Hypercalcemia may be the cause for some of the disturbances of the CNS, including mental aberrations, fatigability, weakness, parasthesias, and headaches. Hypercalcemia may also account for constipation and anorexia. The exact mechanism for the peptic ulceration in primary hyperparathyroidism is not known. There is some evidence, however, that it may be associated with hypercalcemia rather than with PTH excess.[70,71] First, there is usually a significant hypercalcemia among patients with primary hyperparathyroidism suffering from peptic ulceration. It is very uncommon among patients whose serum Ca is only slightly elevated or within the normal range. Second, hypercalcemia itself, rather than PTH excess, is associated with hypersecretion of gastrin and hydrochloric acid.[70,71] This explanation is inadequate, however, since not all patients with primary hyperparathyroidism demonstrate gastric acid hypersecretion despite hypercalcemia. Moreover, hypercalcemia may cause polyuria by impairing renal concentrating ability[72] and by increasing solute load.

The cause for the hypertension in primary hyperparathyroidism is not known. It may be partly the result of hypercalcemia, since an induced hypercalcemia in susceptible individuals may provoke hypertension.[73] Parathyroidectomy often may not restore normal blood pressure, however, even though hypertension may be more easily controlled.[5,6,74,75]

Clinical Presentation of Primary Hyperparathyroidism

Nephrolithiasis, bone disease, and peptic ulcer disease represent symptoms commonly associated with primary hyperparathyroidism. When one or more of the triad is present in patients with hypercalcemia, a vigorous search for primary hyperparathyroidism should be conducted. Less specific symptoms, present particularly in patients with significant hypercalcemia, include mental aberrations, fatigability, weakness, parasthesias, headache, constipation, anorexia, and polyuria.

The clinical presentation of primary hyperparathyroidism may take three general patterns: (1) In patients presenting principally with osteitis fibrosa, the disease is usually of short duration and the degree of hypercalcemia may be marked. Nephrolithiasis is uncommon. (2) In contrast, patients with nephrolithiasis tend to have less severe hypercalcemia and longer duration of the disease. (3) The third group of patients may have no symptoms attributable to the disease or to hypercalcemia. These presentations were considered to be points on the same continuum, reflecting varying severity of PTH excess.[4] Thus, parathyroid glandular size (which may be reflected in degree of PTH secretion) was found to be significantly greater in patients with osteitis than in patients presenting principally with nephrolithiasis.[45] The separation among the three groups is not sharply demarcated, however, since many patients may not fit into any of these patterns. Moreover, the extent of physiological derangements, e.g., hypercalciuria and negative Ca balance, was found to be just as severe in some patients with asymptomatic primary hyperparathyroidism as in their symptomatic counterparts.[76]

Changing Trend in Clinical Presentation

There has been a dramatic change in the clinical presentation of primary hyperparathyroidism since the introduction of the systematic analysis of serum calcium (e.g., SMA).[2] The study of Cope[1] in 1966 probably reflects the situation during the "pre-SMA" era. Nephrolithiasis was the most frequent complication occurring in 57%. Bone disease was present in 23%, and peptic ulceration in 8%. A lump in the neck, later identified as parathyroid adenoma, was the presenting symptom in one of 343 cases. It is indeed an infrequent finding. If a mass is palpated in the neck, it must be presumed to be thyroid unless proved otherwise. In this series, only 2 of 343 cases (1%) were considered to be asymptomatic, and only 6 (2%) had hypertension.

Since the introduction of routine analysis of serum Ca, typical symptomatology of primary hyperparathyroidism continues to be nephrolithiasis, bone disease, and peptic ulcer disease. The occur-

TABLE VI. Clinical Presentation of Primary Hyperparathyroidism[a]

Presenting feature	Cope[1] (N = 343)	Bone et al.[2] (N = 79)
Overt bone disease	23	14
Nephrolithiasis	57	32
Peptic ulcer disease	8	9
Hypertension	2	43
Asymptomatic	1	20

[a] Results expressed as percentages of total cases.

rence of hypertension, however, has become more prominent, and the percentage of those who are aysmptomatic has increased dramatically (Table VI). In our series,[2] 43% of cases had hypertension and 20% of patients were asymptomatic. Other series have reported similar findings.[3,4,74,77] The increased frequency of asymptomatic primary hyperparathyroidism probably reflects improved methods for the assessment of parathyroid function and earlier disclosure through the routine analysis of serum Ca.

The changing trend in the clinical presentation of primary hyperparathyroidism has presented new diagnostic and therapeutic challenges. The diagnosis of primary hyperparathyroidism may be difficult in certain asymptomatic patients in whom the hyperparathyroid state may not be fully manifested. Moreover, a better definition of indications for parathyroidectomy would seem to be warranted in asymptomatic primary hyperparathyroidism.

Diagnosis of Primary Hyperparathyroidism

Various biochemical presentations of primary hyperparathyroidism were discussed in Chapter 3.

Biochemically, the diagnosis of primary hyperparathyroidism may be made from determinations of serum Ca, P, iPTH,[11,78,79] and urinary cAMP.[11,13,80-82] Serum Ca is almost always elevated, but is seldom greater than 14 mg%. When it is normal, it may be increased above normal by certain provocative procedures, such as oral administration of thiazide[83,84] or P-binding antacids.[85] For example, primary hyperparathyroidism should be suspected if the serum Ca concentration exceeds 11 mg% after 2 weeks of treatment with hydrochlorothiazide (50 mg twice a day). Serum P is sometimes low, but is usually within the normal range. The immunoassay for serum PTH may be very helpful, particularly when the antiserum directed against the carboxyterminal end of the PTH molecule is utilized and the values for iPTH are corrected for serum Ca.[79] Since PTH provides a potent stimulus to the renal adenyl cyclase,[86] urinary cAMP may be significantly elevated in primary hyperparathyroidism.[11,13,80-82] A positive correlation between urinary cAMP and serum iPTH has been reported.[4,11] When it is obtained from urine samples collected for 24 hr under controlled diet and environment, it may provide an "integrated" measure of parathyroid function.[11] Urinary cAMP measured in spot random samples has a limited value because of marked circadian variation,[13,80] despite contention to the contrary.[81]

Urinary cAMP may be normal despite parathyroid stimulation in renal disease (glomerular filtration rate < 40 ml/min). It may be elevated in certain conditions other than primary hyperparathyroidism, such as diabetes mellitus,[87] pheochromocytoma,[88] excessive secretion of antidiuretic hormone,[89] thyrotoxicosis,[90] and secondary hyperparathyroidism of renal hypercalciuria[13] and osteomalacia.[91] Recent studies indicate that the determination of "nephrogenous" cAMP (exclusive of filtered component) may yield a better measure of parathyroid function.[92] It may be useful in excluding certain conditions in which the increased urinary cAMP is the result of non-PTH-dependent, extrarenal stimulation of adenyl cyclase.

The serum chloride/phosphorus (Cl/P) ratio, though increased in some cases of primary hyperparathyroidism,[93-95] has a limited value because of the wide overlap into the control range.[96]

The measurement of iPTH in samples of venous blood draining parathyroid glands may help localize the site of abnormal parathyroid tissue. This technique is particularly useful in recurrent primary hyperparathyroidism or in patients who have had neck surgery.[4]

Indications for Parathyroidectomy

The need for parathyroidectomy in symptomatic primary hyperparathyroidism is well recognized. Following removal of abnormal parathyroid tissue, stone formation may cease or decrease in frequency.[7] As discussed earlier, parathyroidectomy decreases urinary Ca and the APR (state of saturation) and increases the FPR (limit of metastability of brushite and Ca oxalate). Moreover, parathyroid surgery usually causes healing of bone, an improvement in peptic ulcer disease, and amelioration of other less specific symptoms of primary hyperparathyroidism.

The efficacy of parathyroidectomy in asymptomatic primary hyperparathyroidism is more difficult to establish. There is considerable controversy as to whether asymptomatic patients should undergo parathyroidectomy. Purnell et al.[3] found that only 9% of asymptomatic patients progressed to meet their criteria for parathyroidectomy over the ensuing 5 years. Williamson and Van-Peenen[97] felt that little is to be gained by diagnosing and treating mild hyperparathyroidism. Hellstrom and Ivemark,[98] however, recommended parathyroidectomy as soon as the diagnosis of primary hyperparathyroidism was made.

Recent studies[9,76] indicate that there may be major physiological derangements indicative of PTH excess in patients with primary hyperparathyroidism even though they may be asymptomatic. These derangements include hypercalciuria, (urinary Ca > 200 mg/day on a diet containing 400 mg Ca and 100 meq Na/day), which predisposes to nephrolithiasis; evidence for negative Ca balance, which may be demonstrated by high fasting urinary Ca, urinary Ca exceeding absorbed Ca, and low bone density; and reduced endogenous creatinine clearance of less than 65 ml/min. These "deleterious sequelae of PTH excess" may be restored toward normal following parathyroidectomy. Thus, parathyroidectomy may be indicated in asymptomatic primary hyperparathyroidism if these physiological derangements are present.

Certain patients with asymptomatic primary hyperparathyroidism may not present physiological derangements; i.e., they may have normal urinary Ca, bone density, and creatinine clearance, and may not be in negative Ca balance.[99] Some progress to develop these derangements or become symptomatic. A significant portion, however, continue to be without physiological derangements.[99] Parathyroidectomy might be withheld in such patients if they could be followed carefully. More experience is required before a more firm recommendation can be made regarding the disposition of patients with asymptomatic primary hyperparathyroidism.

There is no effective medical treatment for the nephrolithiasis of primary hyperparathyroidism.

NORMOCALCEMIC PRIMARY HYPERPARATHYROIDISM

Classically, the diagnosis of primary hyperparathyroidism has required the demonstration of an elevated serum concentration of Ca.[100,101] It has been reported, however, that some patients with primary hyperparathyroidism may present with normal serum Ca concentration.[7,9,14-16] The existence of such "normocalcemic" primary hyperparathyroidism has been questioned, because clear-cut biochemical or histological evidence has sometimes been lacking.[7,102] The features of this condition are: (1) normocalcemia; (2) biochemical evidence of hyperparathyroidism, as indicated by high serum iPTH and urinary cAMP,[9] or by an abnormal response to an intravenous infusion of Ca,[103] or by both; (3) hypercalciuria; (4) state of negative Ca balance, with urinary Ca greater than the absorbed Ca[9]; (5) recurrent Ca urolithiasis as the only recognized clinical symptomatology; (6) histological demonstration of hyperplastic or adenomatous parathyroid glands, even in the absence of gross glandular enlargement[7,14]; and (8) objective and subjective improvement after parathyroidectomy, with correction of biochemical abnormalities (including hypercalciuria) and an improvement in stone disease.[7,104]

Three pathogenetic mechanisms have been proposed for this condition. First, it hs been suggested that normocalcemic primary hyperparathyroidism represents the sequelae of an elaboration in excessive amounts of "atypical" PTH or of calcitonin, which is secreted in response to PTH excess.[37] Hypercalciuria may then be explained by the direct renal effect of calcitonin or by the inability of the atypical PTH to agument renal tubular reabsorption of Ca. Moreover, calcitonin excess could account for the failure of development of significant hypercalcemia or of bone disease. However, biochemical evidence for this hypothesis is totally lacking. The demonstration of increased serum iPTH and urinary cAMP[9] suggests that the PTH elaborated may not be immunologically or biologically dissimilar.

Second, normocalcemic primary hyperparathyroidism may represent an early or a mild form of primary hyperparathyroidism. This hypothesis is supported by the observation that the serum Ca concentration may be intermittently elevated or is in the upper range of normal. Even though the initial serum Ca concentration may be within the normal range, it usually decreases following parathyroid operation.[7] The correction of hypercalciuria could therefore be explained simply from the decrease in the filtered load of Ca. This hypothesis emphasizes the impreciseness of total serum Ca concentration in the diagnosis of mild forms of primary hyperparathyroidism.

The final mechanism implicates this condition as the "end-stage" of renal hypercalciuria.[10,11,13] This hypothesis assumes that PTH secretion may become "autonomous," from a prolonged stimulation of parathyroid glands by the renal leak of Ca. The frequent demonstration of hyperplastic parathyroid glands supports this hypothesis. The correction of hypercalciuria following parathyroidectomy argues against this scheme, however, since persistent hypercalciuria would have been expected if the renal leak of Ca were present. Nevertheless, this form of presentation could occur, though infrequently, as illustrated by the following case.

Case 3. A 55-year-old black woman was referred for parathyroidectomy. She had a history of recurrent passage of Ca-containing renal stones since she was 30 years old. Previous evaluations had disclosed normocalcemia and hypercalciuria. A metabolic evaluation 3 years before indicated that she was suffering from renal hypercalciuria and secondary hyperparathyroidism.

Serum Ca concentration was 9.8 mg% and serum P 3.2 mg%. Urinary Ca on an intake of 400 mg Ca and 100 meq sodium/day was elevated at 250 mg/day. Fasting urinary Ca was high at 0.17 mg/mg creatinine (upper range of normal: 0.11). Serum iPTH and urinary cAMP were elevated. Thiazide therapy restored normal urinary Ca and parathyroid function without causing a significant increase in serum Ca concentration.[10] Unfortunately, the patient discontinued thiazide therapy after 6 months.

On admission, serum Ca concentration was higher than before, and ranged from 10.1 to 10.7 mg%. Serum P was 2.8 mg%. Urinary Ca was 350 mg/day and fasting urinary Ca was 0.18 mg/mg creatinine. High values of serum iPTH and urinary cAMP were found. During parathyroid exploration, one grossly enlarged gland was resected and was identified histologically as a parathyroid nodular hyperplasia. The biopsy of remaining slightly enlarged glands disclosed parathyroid hyperplasia.

Following parathyroid surgery, serum Ca concentration was 9.5 mg%. She continued to have hypercalciuria of 260 mg/day and high fasting urinary Ca of 0.17 mg/mg creatinine.

In conclusion, the condition of normocalcemic primary hyperparathyroidism with the features described above can best be explained by the second mechanism, which considers it as a less severe form of primary hyperparathyroidism. It should not be confused with renal hypercalciuria[10,11] (Cases 1 and 3). Response to thiazide treatment may differentiate between the two conditions, since the serum Ca concentration may increase significantly in normocalcemic primary hyperparathyroidism,[83,84] unlike in renal hypercalciuria.[10]

OTHER CAUSES OF HYPERCALCEMIA

Nephrolithiasis is relatively uncommon in hypercalcemias other than primary hyperparathyroidism. The following description should be useful in the differential diagnosis of primary hyperparathyroidism (Table VII).

TABLE VII. Differential Diagnosis of Hypercalcemias

	Primary hyperparathyroidism	Ectopic "PTH" production	Ectopic PGE production	OAF production
Renal stones Skeletal fracture Peptic ulcer	Frequent	Rare	Rare	Rare
Weight loss	Rare	Frequent	Frequent	Frequent
Onset	Slow	Rapid	Rapid	Rapid
Localizing symptoms of malignancy	Rare	Frequent	Frequent	Frequent
Carcinoma	Rare	"Solid" > "soft"	"Solid"	"Soft"
Treatment	Parathyroidectomy		Indomethacin aspirin	Steroids
Serum Ca	↑	↑↑	↑↑	↑↑
Serum P	↓, N	↓, N	N	N
Serum Cl	N, ↑	N	N	N
Urinary Ca	↑, N	↑↑	↑↑	↑↑
Serum PTH	↑↑	↑	↓	↓
Urinary cAMP	↑	↑	?	↓

Ectopic Parathyroid Hormone Production

In 1941, Albright[105] first described a case of renal-cell carcinoma with hypercalcemia and hypophosphatemia. The chemical finding of hypercalcemia was reversed by radiotherapy to solitary bone metastasis and reappeared with recurrence of metastasis. He postulated that the neoplastic tissue was producing a substance that was biologically similar to PTH. Thus, the concept of "ectopic PTH production" was introduced several decades before the chemical characterization of PTH. In 1956, Plimpton and Gellhorn[106] reported the case of a 49-year-old man with renal-cell carcinoma with hypercalcemia, in whom nephrectomy restored the serum Ca to normal. Unlike the case of Albright, this patient did not have skeletal metastasis. Since there was no direct destruction of bone to produce the hypercalcemia, this case more clearly documented the humoral etiology for the hypercalcemia. These cases provide a reminder that the presence of osteolytic metastasis need not necessarily exclude a humoral mechanism for the hypercalcemia.

Since then, a wide variety of neoplasias have been associated with ectopic PTH production.[107-110] While most were "solid" tumors, some were "soft" (lymphosarcoma, Hodgkin's disease). Most common were renal-cell carcinoma and squamous-cell carcinoma of the lung.

The hormone production by neoplasia has now been documented by the demonstration of immunoreactive PTH in neoplastic tissue by immunoassay, immunofluorescent localization, and autoradiography.[110,111] The ectopic PTH hormone is probably not identical structurally to the native hormone produced by parathyroid glands, since it has been shown to be less reactive immunologically than the native hormone.[110] The ectopic PTH probably possesses the same biological activity, however, since it promotes bone resorption, causes phosphaturia and hypercalcemia, and probably stimulates renal adenyl cyclase.

The presentation of ectopic PTH production differs from primary hyperparathyroidism in the following respects: (1) the onset of hypercalcemia is much more sudden and progressive; (b) the degree of hypercalcemia and hypercalciuria is more marked, often exceeding 14 mg% and 600 mg/day, respectively; (3) hypophosphatemia is usually present; (d) serum Cl/P is usually less than 33, whereas it may be greater than this value in the majority of cases with primary hyperparathyroidism[93]; (5) symptoms of peptic ulceration, skeletal fractures, and renal stones are usually absent, a situation probably reflecting the acute course of the disease; and (6) serum alkaline phosphatase activity is more frequently elevated.

Treatment usually consists of antitumor therapy and correction of acute hypercalcemia.

Ectopic Prostaglandin Production

In 1960, Goldhaber[112] discovered hypercalcemia in the mouse with fibrosarcoma. The extract of the tumor tissue was found to cause bone resorption in tissue culture. Subsequently, Tashjian et al.[113] demonstrated production of prostaglandin E_2 (PGE_2) by the mouse fibrosarcoma. Inhibition of PGE_2 synthesis by indomethacin restored serum Ca to normal, commensurate with decreased levels of circulating PGE_2. It is now known that PGE_1 and E_2 stimulate skeletal adenyl cyclase and cause bone resorption in vitro.[114]

The possibility that there might be a parallel to this animal model in man was suggested by Powell et al.[115] In tumor extracts of patients with hypercalcemia, these workers found bone-resorbing activity in tissue culture, but no immunoassayable PTH. It is now recognized that certain human neoplasias are capable of producing PGs. PG-like substance and immunoreactive PG (E, A, and F) have been identified in tumor tissue.[116] Elevated levels of immunoreactive PGs in serum[116] and high renal excretion of the major urinary metabolite of PGE have been demonstrated.[117] Treatment with indomethacin or aspirin has been shown to ameliorate hypercalcemia, commensurate with the decline in serum immunoreactive PGs and urinary PG metabolite.[116,117] As in the case of ectopic PTH production, it is reasonable to speculate that PG (probably E) produced by neoplastic tissue is carried via hematogenous circulation to bone, where it stimulates resorption, thereby causing hypercalcemia.

The presentation of ectopic PG production resembles that of ectopic PTH production, with the following exceptions: (1) serum iPTH is suppressed; (2) serum P is usually normal; and (3) it is invariably caused by solid tumors. The renal excretion of cAMP has not been measured, but it may be elevated. Unlike ectopic PTH production, the hypercalcemia of ectopic PG production is responsive to indomethacin or aspirin.

Osteoclast-Activating Factor

In 1971, Raisz became intrigued with the problem of localized resorption of bone associated with chronic inflammation (such as periodontal disease), while he was on a sabbatical leave at the National Institute of Dental Research. He then initiated his classic studies concerned with the delineation of osteoclast-activating factor (OAF). It was found that lymphocytes, upon stimulation by antigens to which the donor has developed cellular immunity or by nonspecific mitogens (solubilized dental plaque or phytohemagglutinin), produce a soluble substance that stimulates bone resorption in organ culture.[118] The substance was termed "osteoclast-activating factor" because the treated bone showed numerous active osteoclasts. The OAF could be distinguished from PTH, PGE_2, and $1\alpha,25$-$(OH)_2D$ from dose–response curves (in terms of ^{47}Ca release from bone).[119] Moreover, OAF-stimulated bone resorption was inhibited more effectively by cortisol than was PTH stimulation. The chemical identification of OAF has not yet been completed.[120]

The clinical importance of OAF was realized when it was shown that this substance could also be produced by neoplastic cells as part of the cellular immune response to neoplasia.[119] Lymphoid cell lines from patients with myeloma, Burkitt's lymphoma, and malignant lymphoma were shown to elaborate OAF. The supernatant fluid from short-term cultures of bone marrow from patients with multiple myeloma was shown to contain OAF.[119] The OAF produced by these soft tumors may cause hypercalcemia by stimulating osteoclastic bone resorption. Unlike the case with ectopic PTH or PG production, the effect of OAF is probably confined to bone. It is probably formed in bone on invasion by tumor, and causes bone destruction locally.

The hypercalcemia from excessive OAF production is resistant to indomethacin, but is probably responsive to adrenal corticosteroids.

Neoplasm with Synthesis of Sterol

It is theoretically possible that hypercalcemia in certain neoplasia is the consequence of increased synthesis of $1\alpha,$ 25-$(OH)_2D$ by the tumor tissue.[121] The vitamin D metabolite may then cause hypercalcemia by promoting skeletal resorption and stimulating intestinal Ca absorption. Although increased synthesis of $1\alpha,25$-$(OH)_2D$ has not yet been demonstrated in any neoplasm, Gordan *et al.* [122] reported the production in breast cancer of a certain sterol that stimulated bone resorption. This sterol has not yet been identified chemically. It is noteworthy that the hypercalcemia of breast cancer is fairly responsive to treatment by adrenal corticosteroids, [123] as in vitamin D intoxication.

The frequency of involvement of various humoral mechanisms (e.g. ectopic PTH or PG, OAF, or sterol) in cancer is not known.

Osteolytic Metastasis

When certain neoplasias invade bone, they may cause hypercalcemia by direct destruction of bone without involving humoral substances. Destruction of only 1% of bone over a 12-day period may be sufficient to cause hypercalcemia in a 70-kg man, since it may release from bone into the circulation more than 800 mg Ca each day. As in ectopic PTH production, serum and urinary Ca may be markedly increased. However, serum P is usually normal and both serum iPTH and urinary cAMP are suppressed. As mentioned above, the presence of osteolytic metastasis need not exclude the operation of humoral mechanisms for the hypercalcemia.

The hypercalcemia of osteolytic metastasis is more responsive to adrenocorticosteroids than that of ectopic PTH or PG production.

Sarcoidosis

Hypercalcemia of sarcoidosis is probably vitamin-D-dependent. [124,125] It may be provoked by low doses of vitamin D, and ameliorated by adrenal corticosteroids as in vitamin D toxicity. Although hypersensitivity to vitamin D has been previously invoked, recent studies suggest that there may be an increased synthesis of $1\alpha,25\text{-}(OH)_2D$. [126] Hypercalcemia is probably the consequence of either vitamin-D-dependent intestinal hyperabsorption of Ca or excessive skeletal Ca mobilization, or both.

Milk–Alkali Syndrome

In 1949, Burnett et al. [127] described hypercalcemia developing following prolonged intake of milk and absorbable alkali. Characteristic features were hypercalcemia without hypophosphatemia, low urinary Ca, mild metabolic alkalosis, normal serum alkaline phosphatase activity, marked renal insufficiency, and calcinosis. Improvement ensued on avoidance of milk and alkali.

The primary pathogenetic event is the absorption of large amounts of Ca and alkali. The ensuing alkalosis promotes renal tubular reabsorption of Ca. Hypercalcemia probably develops from the increased Ca absorption and impaired renal Ca excretion. Renal insufficiency further contributes to hypercalcemia by limiting renal Ca excretion. As might be expected, parathyroid function is suppressed.

It is possible that patients who develop milk–alkali syndrome are probably those who initially had an intestinal hyperabsorption of Ca. This hypothesis could explain the apparent predilection for the syndrome in a minority of cases exposed to excessive milk and alkali ingestion, and correction of hypercalcemia by limitation of intestinal Ca absorption with cellulose phosphate.

The situation in milk–alkali syndrome contrasts strikingly with that in absorptive hypercalciuria,[11] in which hypercalcemia rarely develops despite intestinal hyperabsorption of Ca. The results suggest that in the absence of enhanced bone mobilization and defective renal excretion of Ca, the increased delivery of Ca from the intestinal tract may be handled adequately by physiological compensatory mechanisms.

The milk–alkali syndrome has become infrequent with the decreasing popularity of absorbable antacids and with wider usage of nonabsorbable alkali.

Phosphorus-Depletion Syndrome

Nonabsorbable antacids may also cause hypercalcemia by a different mechanism.

Mild hypercalcemia (up to 11 mg%) and marked hypophosphatemia may ensue from dietary P restriction and ingestion of P-binding antacids.[85,128] Urinary Ca is typically high and urinary P unusually low. Parathyroid function is suppressed.

Hypercalcemia is partly the consequence of an increased intestinal Ca absorption. Although the synthesis of $1\alpha,25$-$(OH)_2D$ has been shown to be stimulated in hypophosphatemic experimental animals,[129] there is no evidence that the circulating concentration of $1\alpha,25$-$(OH)_2D$ is altered by P deprivation in man. On the other hand, P deprivation may increase the available Ca for absorption, by limiting the amount of intraluminal phosphate. Thus, the increased Ca absorption occurring in P deprivation in man may be at least in part the result of an increased available Ca pool. The enhanced mobilization of Ca from bone, associated with hypophosphatemia,[130] probably contributes to the development of hypercalcemia.

Thiazide Therapy

Thiazide is unique among diuretics in stimulating renal tubular reabsorption of Ca[10,83,131,132] (see Chapter 3 for a discussion of the mechanism). Although it was believed to stimulate bone resorption via parathyroid glands,[133] conclusive evidence for this contention is lacking. Thiazide effect on intestinal Ca absorption has not been clearly defined. In normal man, the intestinal Ca absorption is not altered or is slightly increased during treatment.

Mild hypercalcemia (up to 10.6 mg%) may ensue during thiazide therapy in normal man.[83] Part of this rise in serum Ca probably reflects the increased protein-bound Ca; the reduction in extracellular fluid volume augments the circulating concentration of proteins and probably causes increased Ca binding. The circulating Ca^{2+} is probably also increased slightly through the inhibition of renal Ca loss. The latter mechanism may be predominant in conditions characterized by an excessive skeletal mobilization of Ca,[84] such as primary hyperparathyroidism. Under such circumstances, true hypercalcemia, reflected by a rise in plasma Ca^{2+}, may be found. The total serum Ca may reach moderately high levels.

REFERENCES

1. Cope, O. 1966. The story of hyperparathyroidism at the Massachusetts General Hospital. *N. Engl. J. Med.* **274:**1174–1182.
2. Bone, H. G., III, Snyder, W. H., III, and Pak, C. Y. C. 1977. Diagnosis of hyperparathyroidism. *Annu. Rev. Med.* **28:**111–117.
3. Purnell, D. C., Smith, L. H., Scholz, D. A., Elveback, L. R., and Arnaud, C. D. 1971. Primary hyperparathyroidism: A prospective clinical study. *Am. J. Med.* **50:**670–678.
4. Mallette, L. E., Bilezikian, J. P., Heath, D. A., and Aurbach, G. D. 1974. Primary hyperparathyroidism: Clinical and biochemical features. *Medicine (Baltimore)* **53:**127–146.
5. Watson, L. 1974. Primary hyperparathyroidism. *Clin. Endocrinol. Metab.* **3:**215–235.
6. Myers, R. T. 1974. Followup study of surgically-treated primary hyperparathyroidism. *Ann. Surg.* **179:**729–733.
7. George, J. M., Rabson, A. S., Ketcham, A., and Bartter, F. C. 1965. Calcareous renal disease and hyperparathyroidism. *Q. J. Med.* **64:**291–301.
8. Chalmers, T. M., Adams, P., Adams, J. E., Hill, L. F., Truscott, B. McN., and Smellie, W. A. B. 1972. Normocalcemic primary hyperparathyroidism, idiopathic hypercalciuria and calcium-containing renal stones. In *Extrait du Symposium Rein et Calcium*. Sandoz, pp. 295–306.
9. Pak, C. Y. C., East, C., Sanzenbacher, L. J., Delea, C. S., and Bartter, F. C. 1972. Gastrointestinal calcium absorption in nephrolithiasis. *J. Clin. Endocrinol. Metab.* **35:**261–270.
10. Coe, F. L., Canterbury, J. M., Firpo, J. J., and Reiss, E. 1973. Evidence for secondary hyperparathyroidism in idiopathic hypercalciuria. *J. Clin. Invest.* **52:**134–142.
11. Pak, C. Y. C., Ohata, M., Lawrence, E. C., and Snyder, W. 1974. The hypercalciurias: Causes, parathyroid functions and diagnostic criteria. *J. Clin. Invest.* **54:**387–400.
12. Nordin, B. E. C., Peacock, M., and Wilkinson, R. 1972. Hypercalciuria and calcium stone disease. In *Clinics in Endocrinology and Metabolism*, Vol. 1, No. 1, I. McIntyre, Ed. W. B. Saunders, Philadelphia, pp. 169–183.
13. Pak, C. Y. C., Kaplan, R. A., Bone, H., Townsend, J., and Waters, O. 1975. A simple test for the diagnosis of absorptive, resorptive and renal hypercalciurias. *N. Engl. J. Med.* **292:**497–500.

14. Wills, M. R., Pak, C. Y. C., Hammond, W. G., and Bartter, F. C. 1969. Normocalcemic primary hyperparathyroidism. *Am. J. Med.* **47**:384–391.
15. Frame, B., Foroozanfar, F., and Patton, R. B. 1970. Normocalcemic primary hyperparathyroidism with osteitis fibrosa. *Ann. Intern. Med.* **73**:253–257.
16. Johnson, R. D., and Conn, J. W. 1969. Hyperparathyroidism with a prolonged period of normocalcemia. *J. Am. Med. Assoc.* **210**:2063–2066.
17. Neuman, W. F., and Neuman, M. W. 1958. *The Chemical Dynamics of Bone Mineral.* University of Chicago Press.
18. Robertson, W. G., Peacock, M., and Nordin, B. E. C. 1968. Activity products in stone-forming and non-stone-forming urine. *Clin. Sci.* **34**:579–594.
19. Finlayson, B., Roth, R., and DuBois, L. 1972. Calcium oxalate solubility studies. In *Urinary Calculi: Proceedings of the International Symposium on Renal Stone Research, Madrid, 1972.* L. Cifuentes Delatte, A. Rapado, and A. Hodgkinson, Eds. Karger, Basel and New York, pp. 1–7.
20. Pak, C. Y. C., Hayashi, Y., Finlayson, B., and Chu, S. 1977. Estimation of the state of saturation of brushite and calcium oxalate in urine: A comparison of three methods. *J. Lab. Clin. Med.* **89**:891–901.
21. Toribara, T. Y. 1953. Centrifuge type of ultrafiltration apparatus. *Anal. Chem.* **25**:1286.
22. Halver, B. 1972. A rapid method for the determination of ultrafiltrable calcium in serum. *Clin. Chem.* **18**:1488–1492.
23. Moore, E. W. 1970. Ionized calcium in normal serum, ultrafiltrates, and whole blood determined by ion-exchange electrodes. *J. Clin. Invest.* **49**:318–334.
24. Orion Research Incorporated. 1975. Model SS-20 Ionized Calcium Analyzer. Brochure.
25. Pak, C. Y. C. 1969. Physicochemical basis for the formation of renal stones of calcium phosphate origin: Calculation of the degree of saturation of urine with respect to brushite. *J. Clin. Invest.* **48**:1914–1922.
26. Sherwood, L. M., Mayer, G. P., Rambery, C. F., Jr., Kronfeld, D. S., Aurbach, G. D., and Potts, J. T., Jr. 1968. Regulation of parathyroid hormone secretion: Proportional control by calcium, lack of effect of phosphate. *Endocrinology* **83**:1043–1051.
27. Raisz, L. G. 1965. Bone resorption in tissue culture: Factors influencing the response to parathyroid hormone. *J. Clin. Invest.* **44**:103–116.
28. Wills, M. R., Wortsman, J., Pak, C. Y. C., and Bartter, F. C. 1970. The role of parathyroid hormone in the gastrointestinal absorption of calcium. *Clin. Sci.* **39**:89–94.
29. Agus, Z. S., Gardner, L. B., Beck, L. H., and Goldberg, M. 1973. Effects of parathyroid hormone on renal tubular reabsorption of calcium, sodium, and phosphate. *Am. J. Physiol.* **224**:1143–1148.
30. DeLuca, H. F. 1975. The kidney as an endocrine organ involved in the function of vitamin D. *Am. J. Med.* **58**:39–47.

31. Omdahl, J., Holick, M., Suda, T., Tanaka, Y., and DeLuca, H. F. 1971. Biological activity of 1,25-dihydroxycholecalciferol. *Biochemistry* **10:**2935–2940.

32. Reynolds, J. J., Holick, M. F., and DeLuca, H. F. 1973. The role of vitamin D metabolites in bone resorption. *Calcif. Tissue Res.* **12:**295–301.

33. Puschett, J. B., Fernandez, P. C., Boyle, J. T., Gray, R. W., Omdahl, J. L., and DeLuca, H. F. 1972. The acute renal tubular effects of 1,25-dihydroxycholecalciferol. *Proc. Soc. Endocrinol. Metab.* **141:**379–384.

34. Garabedian, M., Holick, M. F., DeLuca, H. F., and Boyle, J. T. 1972. Control of 25-hydroxycholecalciferol metabolism by parathyroid glands. *Proc. Natl. Acad. Sci. U.S.A.* **69:**1673–1676.

35. Kaplan, R. A., Haussler, M. R., Deftos, L. J., Bone, H., and Pak, C. Y. C. The role of 1α,25-dihydroxycholecalciferol in the mediation of intestinal hyperabsorption of calcium in primary hyperparathyroidism and absorptive hypercalciuria. *J. Clin. Invest.* **59:**756–760.

36. Raisz, L. G. Au, W. Y. W., Friedman, J., and Niemann, I. 1967. Thyrocalcitonin and bone resorption. *Am. J. Med.* **43:**684–690.

37. Pak, C. Y. C. 1971. Parathyroid hormone and thyrocalcitonin: Their mode of action and regulation. *Ann. N. Y. Acad. Sci.* **179:**450–474.

38. Gray, T. K., Bieberdorf, F. A., and Fordtran, J. S. 1973. Thyrocalcitonin and the jejunal absorption of calcium, water, and electrolytes in normal subjects. *J. Clin. Invest.* **52:**3084–3088.

39. Arnaud, C. D., Tsao, H. S., and Littledike, T. 1970. Calcium homeostasis, parathyroid hormone, and calcitonin: Preliminary report. *Mayo Clin. Proc.* **45:**125–131.

40. Francis, M. D., and Webb, N. C. 1971. Hydroxyapatite formation from a hydrated calcium monohydrogen phosphate precursor. *Calcif. Tissue Res.* **6:**335–342.

41. Pak, C. Y. C. Eanes, E. D., and Ruskin, B. 1971. Spontaneous precipitation of brushite: Evidence that brushite is the nidus of renal stones originating as calcium phosphate. *Proc. Natl. Acad. Sci. U.S.A.* **68:**1456–1460.

42. Nordin, B. E. C., and Peacock, M. 1969. Role of kidney in regulation of plasma-calcium. *Lancet* **2:**1280–283.

43. Keating, R. F., Jones, J. D., Elveback, L. R., and Randall, R. V. 1969. The relation of age and sex to distribution of values in healthy adults of serum calcium, inorganic phosphorus, magnesium, alkaline phosphatase, total proteins, albumin, and blood urea. *J. Lab. Clin. Med.* **73:**825–834.

44. Dauphine, R. T., Riggs, B. L., and Scholz, D. A. 1975. Back pain and vertebral crush fractures: An unemphasized mode of presentation for primary hyperparathyroidism. *Ann. Intern. Med.* **83:**365–367.

45. Lloyd, H. M. 1968. Primary hyperparathyroidism: An analysis of the role of the parathyroid tumor. *Medicine (Baltimore)* **47:**53–71.

46. Pak, C. Y. C., and Bartter, F. C. 1972. Treatment of osteoporosis with calcium infusions. *Semin. Drug Treat.* **2:**39–46.

47. Berlyne, G. M., Ben-Ari, J., Galinsky, D., Hirsch, M., Kushelevsky, A., and Shainkin, R. 1974. The etiology of osteoporosis: The role of parathyroid hormone. *J. Am. Med. Assoc.* **229:**1904–1905.

48. Hossain, M., Smith, D. A., and Nordin, B. E. C. 1970. Parathyroid activity and postmenopausal osteoporosis. *Lancet* **1:**809–811.

49. Burkhart, J. M., and Jowsey, J. 1967. Parathyroid and thyroid hormones in the development of immobilization osteoporosis. *Endocrinology* **81:**1053–1062.

50. Jowsey, J., and Raisz, L. G. 1968. Experimental osteoporosis and parathyroid activity. *Endocrinology* **82:**384–396.

51. Henneman, D. H., Pak, C. Y. C., Bartter, F. C., Lifschitz, M. D., and Sanzenbacher, L. 1972. The solubility and synthetic rate of bone collagen in idiopathic osteoporosis. *Clin. Orthop,. Relat. Res.* **88:**275–282.

52. Flanagan, B., and Nichols, G., Jr. 1965. Metabolic studies of human bone *in vitro.* II. Changes in hyperparathyroidism. *J. Clin. Invest.* **44:**1795–1804.

53. Atkins, D., Zanelli, J. M., Peacock, M., and Nordin, B. E. C. 1972. The effect of oestrogens on the response of bone to parathyroid hormone *in vitro. J. Endocrinol.* **54:**107–117.

54. Orimo, H., Fujita, T., and Yoshikawa, M. 1972. Increased sensitivity of bone to parathyroid hormone in ovariectomized rats. *Endocrinology* **90:**760–763.

55. Aitken, J. M., Hart, D. M., and Lindsay, R. 1973. Oestrogen replacement therapy for prevention of osteoporosis after oophorectomy. *Br. Med. J.* **3:**515–518.

56. Dequeker, J. 1972. Treatment with oestrogens of primary hyperparathyroidism in post-menopausal women. *Lancet* **1:**747.

57. Pak, C. Y. C., Stewart, A., Kaplan, R., Bone, H., Notz, C., and Browne, R. 1975. Photon absorptiometric analysis of bone density in primary hyperparathyroidism. *Lancet* **2:**7–9.

58. Gallagher, J. C., Riggs, B. L., Eisman, J., Arnaud, S. B., and DeLuca, H. F. 1976. Impaired production of 1,25-dihydroxy-vitamin D in postmenopausal osteoporosis. *Clin. Res.* **24:**580A.

59. Caputo, C. B., Meadows, D., and Raisz, L. G. Failure of estrogens and androgens to inhibit bone resorption in tissue culture. Submitted for publication.

60. Nordin, B. E. C. 1960. The effect of intravenous parathyroid extract on urinary pH, bicarbonate and electrolyte excretion. *Clin. Sci.* 19:311–319.

61. Massry, S. G. 1977. Metabolic acidosis in hyperparathyroidism: Role of phosphate depletion and other factors. In *Advances in Experimental Medicine and Biology, Vol. 81: Phosphate Metabolism.* S. G. Massry and E. Ritz, Eds. Plenum, New York, pp. 301–307.

62. Pak, C. Y. C., and Holt, K. 1976. Nucleation and growth of brushite and calcium oxalate in urine of stone-formers. *Metabolism* **25:**665–673.

63. Hodgkinson, A., and Pyrah, L. N. 1958. The urinary excretion of calcium

and inorganic phosphate in 344 patients with calcium stones of renal origin. *Br. J. Surg.* **46:**10–18.

64. Pak, C. Y. C. 1972. Nephrolithiasis (Ca-containing). *Acta Endocrinol. Panam.* **3:**45–52.

65. Pak, C. Y. C., and Arnold, L. H. 1975. Heterogeneous nucleation of calcium oxalate by seeds of monosodium urate. *Proc. Soc. Exp. Biol. Med.* **149:**930–932.

66. Pak, C. Y. C., Hayashi, Y., and Arnold, L. H. 1976. Heterogeneous nucleation between urate, calcium phosphate and calcium oxalate. *Proc. Soc. Exp. Biol. Med.* **153:**83–87.

67. Coe, F. L., Lawton, R. L., Goldstein, R. B., and Tembe, V. 1975. Sodium urate accelerates precipitation of calcium oxalate *in vitro*. *Proc. Soc. Exp. Biol. Med.* **149:**926–929.

68. Avioli, L. V., McDonald, J. E., and Singer, R. A. 1965. Excretion of pyrophosphate in disorders of bone metabolism. *J. Clin. Endocrinol. Metab.* **25:**912–915.

69. Russell, R. G. G., and Hodgkinson, A. 1969. The urinary excretion of inorganic pyrophosphate in hyperparathyroidism, hyperthyroidism, Paget's disease and other disorders of bone metabolism. *Clin. Sci.* **36:**435–443.

70. Barreras, R. F. 1973. Calcium and gastric secretion. *Gastroenterology* **64:**1168–1184.

71. Trudeau, W. L., and McGuigan, J. E. 1969. Effects of calcium on serum gastrin levels in the Zollinger–Ellison syndrome. *N. Engl. J. Med.* **281:**862–866.

72. Lindeman, R. D., Adler, S., Yiengst, M. J., and Beard, E. S. 1967. The influence of various nutrients on urinary divalent cation excretion. *J. Lab. Clin. Med.* **70:**236–245.

75. Lifschitz, M. D., Pak, C. Y. C., Henneman, D., Jowsey, J., Pilch, Y., and Bartter, F. C. 1970. Treatment of osteoporosis with calcium infusions. *Trans. Assoc. Am. Physicians* **83:**254–266.

74. Pratley, S. K., Posen, S., and Reeve, T. S. 1973. Primary hyperparathyroidism: Experiences with 60 patients. *Med. J. Aust.* **1:**421–426.

75. Irvin, G. L., III, Cohen, M. S., Moebus, R., and Mintz, D. H. 1972. Primary hyperparathyroidism. *Arch. Surg.* **105:**738–740.

76. Kaplan, R. A., Snyder, W. H., Stewart, A., and Pak, C. Y. C. 1976. Metabolic effects of parathyroidectomy in asymptomic primary hyperparathyroidism. *J. Clin. Endocrinol. Metab.* **42:**415–426.

77. Boonstra, C. E., and Jackson, C. E. 1963. Hyperparathyroidism detected by routine serum calcium analysis: Prevalence in a clinic population. *Ann. Intern. Med.* **63:**468–474.

78. Reiss, E., and Canterbury, J. M. 1971. Genesis of hyperparathyroidism. *Am. J. Med.* **50:**679–685.

79. Arnaud, C. D., Tsao, H. S., and Littledike, T. 1971. Radio-immunoassay of human parathyroid hormone in serum. *J. Clin. Invest.* **50:**21–34.

80. Murad, F., and Pak, C. Y. C. 1972. Urinary excretion of adenosine 3',5'-monophosphate and guanosine 3',5'-monophosphate. *N. Engl. J. Med.* **286:**1382–1387.

81. Shaw, J. W., Oldham, S. B., Rosoff, L., Bethune, J. E., and Fichman, M. P. 1977. Urinary cyclic AMP analyzed as a function of the serum calcium and parathyroid hormone in the differential diagnosis of hypercalcemia. *J. Clin. Invest.* **59:**14–21.

82. Neelon, F. A., Drezner, M., Birch, B. M., and Lebovitz, H. E. 1973. Urinary cyclic adenosine monophosphate as an aid in the diagnosis of hyperparathyroidism. *Lancet* **1:**631–634.

83. Brickman, A. S., Massry, S. G., and Coburn, J. W. 1972. Changes in serum and urinary calcium during treatment with hydrochlorothiazide studies on mechanisms. *J. Clin. Invest.* **51:**945–954.

84. Parfitt, A. M. 1969. Chlorothiazide-induced hypercalcemia in juvenile osteoporosis and hyperparathyroidism. *N. Engl. J. Med.* **281:**55–59.

85. Pronove, P., Bell, N. H., and Bartter, F. C. 1961. Production of hypercalciuria by phosphorus deprivation on a low calcium intake: A new clinical test for hyperparathyroidism. *Metabolism* **10:**364–370.

86. Chase, L. R., and Aurbach, G. D. 1968. Renal adenyl cyclase: Anatomically separate sites for parathyroid hormone and vasopressin. *Science* **159:**545–547.

87. Tucci, J. R., Lin, T., and Kopp, L. 1973. Urinary cyclic 3',5'-adenosine monophosphate levels in diabetes mellitus before and after treatment. *J. Clin. Endocrinol. Metab.* **37:**832–835.

88. Ball, J. H., Kaminsky, N. I., Hardman, J. G., Broadus, A. E., Sutherland, E. W., and Liddle, G. W. 1972. Effects of catecholamines and adrenergic-blocking agents on plasma and urinary cyclic nucleotides in man. *J. Clin. Invest.* **51:**2124–2129.

89. Chase, L. R., and Aurbach, G. D. 1968. Renal adenyl cyclase: Anatomically separate sites for parathyroid hormone and vasopressin. *Science* **159:**545–547.

90. Lin, T., Kopp, L. E., and Tucci, J. R. 1973. Urinary excretion of cyclic-3',5'-adenosine monophosphate in hyperthyroidism. *J. Clin. Endocrinol. Metab.* **36:**1033–1036.

91. Schmidt-Gayk, H., Seitz, H., Stengel, R., and Ritz, E. 1975. Secondary hyperparathyroidism of gastrointestinal and renal origin: Influence of renal function on urinary cyclic AMP. In *12th International Congress of Internal Medicine,* Tel Aviv, 1974. Karger, Basel, pp. 130–134.

92. Babka, J. C., Bower, R. H., and Sode, J. 1976. Nephrogenous cyclic AMP levels in primary hyperparathyroidism. *Arch. Intern. Med.* **136:**1140–1144.

93. Palmer, F. J., Nelson, J. C., and Bacchus, H. 1974. The chloride–phosphate ratio in hypercalcemia. *Ann. Intern. Med.* **80:**200–204.

94. Reeves, C. D., Palmer, F., Bacchus, H., and Longerbeam, J. K. 1975. Dif-

ferential diagnosis of hypercalcemia by the chloride/phosphate ratio. *Am. J. Surg.* **130:**166–171.

95. Drago, J. R., Rohner T. J., Sanford, E. J., and Santen, R. E. 1976. Diagnosis of hyperparathyroidism. *Urology* **7:**4–6.

96. Pak, C. Y. C., and Townsend, J. 1976. Chloride:phosphorus in primary hyperparathyroidism. *Ann. Intern. Med.* **85:**830.

97. Williamson, E., and VanPeenen, 1974. Patient benefit in discovering occult hyperparathyroidism. *Arch. Intern. Med.* **133:**430–431.

98. Hellstrom, J., and Ivemark, B. I. 1962. Primary hyperparathyroidism: Clinical and structural findings in 138 cases. *Acta Chir. Scand. (Suppl.)* **294:**1–113.

99. Barilla, D. E., and Pak, C. Y. C. In preparation.

100. Dent, C. E. 1962. Some problems of hyperparathyroidism. *Br. Med. J.* **2:**1419–1425.

101. Pyrah, L. N., Hodgkinson, A., and Anderson, C. K. 1966. Primary hyperparathyroidism: A critical review. *Br. J. Surg.* **53:**245–316.

102. Roth, S. I. 1962. Pathology of the parathyroid in hyperparathyroidism. *Arch. Pathol.* **73:**495–510.

103. Pak, C. Y. C., East, D., Sanzenbacher, L., Ruskin, B. S., and Cox, J. 1972. A simple and reliable test for the diagnosis of hyperparathyroidism. *Arch. Intern. Med.* **129:**48–55.

104. Sanzenbacher, L. J., East, D. A., Pak, C. Y. C., and Bartter, F. C. 1970. Pre- and post-operative evaluation of patients with normocalcemic primary hyperparathyroidism. *Surg. Forum*, pp. 96–98.

105. Albright, F. 1941. Case records of the Massachusetts General Hospital (Case 27461). *N. Engl. J. Med.* **225:**789–791.

106. Plimpton, C. H., and Gellhorn, A. 1956. Hypercalcemia in malignant disease without evidence of bone destruction. *Am. J. Med.* **21:**750–759.

107. Omenn, G. S., Roth, S. I., and Baker, W. H. 1969. Hyperparathyroidism associated with malignant tumors of nonparathyroid origin. *Cancer* **24:**1004–1012.

108. Lafferty, F. W. 1966. Pseudohyperparathyroidism. *Medicine (Baltimore)* **45:**247–260.

109. Snedecor, P. A., and Baker, H. W. 1964. Pseudohyperparathyroidism due to malignant tumors. *Cancer* **17:**1492–1496.

110. Riggs, B. L., Arnaud, C. D., Reynolds, J. C., and Smith, L. H. 1971. Immunologic differentiation of primary hyperparathyroidism from hyperparathyroidism due to nonparathyroid cancer. *J. Clin. Invest.* **50:**2079–2083.

111. Palmieri, G. M. A., Nordquist, R. E., and Omenn, G. S. 1974. Immunochemical localization of parathyroid hormone in cancer tissue from patients with ectopic hyperparathyroidism. *J. Clin. Invest.* **53:**1726–1735.

112. Goldhaber, P. 1960. Enhancement of bone resorption in tissue culture by mouse fibrosarcoma. *Proc. Am. Assoc. Cancer Res.* **3:**113.

113. Tashjian, A. H., Jr., Voelkel, E. F., Levine, L., and Goldhaber, P. 1972. Evidence that the bone resorption-stimulating factor produced by mouse fibrosarcoma cells is prostaglandin E_2: A new model for the hypercalcemia of cancer. *J. Exp. Med.* **136:**1329–1343.

114. Klein, D. C., and Raisz, L. G. 1970. Prostaglandins: Stimulation of bone resorption in tissue culture. *Endocrinology* **86:**1436–1440.

115. Powell, D., Singer, F. R., Murray, T. M., Minkin, C., and Potts, J. T., Jr. 1973. Nonparathyroid humoral hypercalcemia in patients with neoplastic diseases. *N. Engl. J. Med.* **289:**176–181.

116. Robertson, R. P., Baylink, D. J., Marini, J. J., and Adkison, H. W. 1975. Elevated prostaglandins and suppressed parathyroid hormone associated with hypercalcemia and renal cell carcinoma. *J. Clin. Endocrinol. Metab.* **41:**164–167.

117. Seyberth, H. W., Segre, G. V., Morgan, J. L., Sweetman, B. J., Potts, J. T., Jr., and Oates, J. A. 1975. Prostaglandins as mediators of hypercalcemia associated with certain types of cancer. *N. Engl. J. Med.* **293:**1278–1283.

118. Horton, J. E., Raisz, L. G., Simmons, H. A., Oppenheim, J. J., and Mergenhagen, S. E. 1972. Bone resorbing activity in supernatant fluid from cultured human peripheral blood leukocytes. *Science* **177:**793–795.

119. Mundy, G. R., Luben, R. A., Raisz, L. G., Oppenheim, J. J., and Buell, D. N. 1974. Bone-resorbing activity in supernatants from lymphoid cell lines. *N. Engl. J. Med.* **290:**867–871.

120. Luben, R. A., Mundy, G. R., Trummel, C. L., and Raisz, L. G. 1974. Partial purification of osteoclast-activating factor from phytohemagglutinin-stimulated leukocytes. *J. Clin. Invest.* **53:**1473–1480.

121. Raisz, L. G. 1973. Prostaglandins and the hypercalcemia of cancer. *N. Engl. J. Med.* **289:**214–215.

122. Gordan, G. S., Cantino, T. J., Erhardt, L., Hansen, J., and Lubich, W. 1966. Osteolytic sterol in human breast cancer. *Science* **151:**1226–1228.

123. Davis, H. L., Wiseley, A. N., Ramirez, G., and Ansfield, F. J. 1973. Hypercalcemia complicating breast cancer. *Oncology* **28:**126–137.

124. Bell, N. H., Gill, J. R., Jr., and Bartter, F. C. 1964. On the abnormal calcium absorption in sarcoidosis. *Am. J. Med.* **36:**500–513.

125. Bell, N. H., and Bartter, F. C. 1964. Transient reversal of hyperabsorption of calcium and of abnormal sensitivity to vitamin D in a patient with sarcoidosis during episode of nephritis. *Ann. Intern. Med.* **61:**702–710.

126. Bell, N. H., Sinha, T. K., and DeLuca, H. F. 1976. Mechanism for abnormal calcium metabolism in sarcoidosis. *Clin. Res.* **24:**484.

127. Burnett, C. H., Commons, R. R., Albright, F., and Howard, J. E. 1949. Hypercalcemia without hypercalciuria or hypophosphatemia, calcinosis and renal insufficiency. *N. Engl. J. Med.* **240:**787–794.

128. Lotz, M., Zisman, E., and Bartter, F. C. 1968. Evidence for a phosphorus depletion syndrome in man. *N. Engl. J. Med.* **278:**409–415.

129. Huges, M. R., Brumbaugh, P. F., Haussler, M. R., Wergedal, J. E., and Baylink, D. J. 1975. Regulation of serum 1α,25-dihydroxyvitamin D_3 by calcium and phosphate in the rat. *Science* **190**:578–580.
130. Bruin, W. J., Baylink, D. J., and Wergedal, J. E. 1975. Acute inhibition of mineralization and stimulation of bone resorption mediated by hypophosphatemia. *Endocrinology* **96**:394–399.
131. Middler, S., Pak, C. Y. C., Murad, F., and Bartter, F. C. 1973. Thiazide diuretics and calcium metabolism. *Metabolism* **22**:139–146.
132. Garcia, D. A., and Yendt, E. R. 1970. The effects of probenecid and thiazides and their combination on the urinary excretion of electrolytes and on acid–base equilibrium *Can. Med. Assoc. J.* **103**:473–483.
133. Pickelman, J., Paloyan, E., Forland, M., and Strauss, F. H. 1968. Thiazide induced parathyroid stimulation. *Clin. Res.* **16**:468.

Chapter 5

Hyperuricosuric Calcium Urolithiasis

The term "normocalciuric nephrolithiasis"[1] was initially used to describe patients with recurrent Ca urolithiasis in whom a 24-hr urinary Ca was within the normal range. This condition may be subdivided into the different groups listed in Table VIII. Absorptive hypercalciuria Type II was discussed in Chapter 3. Hyperoxaluria will be covered in Chapter 6. The idiopathic group comprises those patients in whom there is no obvious abnormality for stone formation. Some of these patients give a history of low fluid intake. In others, the formation product ratios (FPRs) (limit of metastability) of brushite and Ca oxalate in urine may be significantly reduced.[2] Thus, urinary supersaturation with respect to Ca salts, resulting from the passage of concentrated urine, and deficiency of inhibitors or presence of promoters of nucleation, or both, may be etiologically important in stone formation in the idiopathic group. This chapter will focus principally on Ca stone formation associated with hyperuricosuria.

HISTORICAL BACKGROUND

Abnormalities in uric acid metabolism have long been recognized in Ca urolithiasis. Certain patients with gout develop renal

TABLE VIII. Classification of
Normocalciuric Calcium Urolithiasis

1. Absorptive hypercalciuria Type II
2. Hyperuricosuric Ca urolithiasis
3. Hyperoxaluria, renal tubular acidosis, infection
4. Idiopathic

stones of Ca oxalate rather than of uric acid.[3,4] In "idiopathic hypercalciuria"[5] and in primary hyperparathyroidism, an increased incidence of hyperuricemia or hyperuricosuria or both has been reported.[6,7]

Hyperuricosuria may also be present as the only discernible abnormality in patients with normocalciuria and recurrent Ca urolithiasis.[6,8,9] The clinical spectrum of this disorder, which this chapter will consider, has gradually evolved, largely through the work of Coe et al.[6,8] First, the patients suffer from recurrent passage of Ca-containing renal stones, composed principally of Ca oxalate. Second, they have normocalciuria and do not present any obvious abnormality of Ca metabolism. Third, they have a persistent hyperuricosuria. The cause of the high renal excretion of uric acid is believed to be dietary overindulgence in purine-rich foods in the majority of cases.[8] Diet history may disclose a higher purine intake than in control subjects. Endogenous overproduction may be present in some cases, since hyperuricosuria may not be eliminated by purine deprivation.[6,10] Fourth, urinary pH is invariably greater than 5.5, unlike the case in patients with gout and uric acid stones, in whom urinary pH is usually less than 5.5. There is probably no defect in renal acidification, however, since urinary pH is not significantly different from that of control subjects maintained on a similar diet. Finally, the treatment with allopurinol has been reported to decrease the frequency of stone formation, commensurate with the reduction in renal excretion of uric acid.[6,8,11]

CAUSE OF CALCIUM UROLITHIASIS IN HYPERURICOSURIA

In patients with hyperuricosuric Ca urolithiasis with normocalciuria, the high renal excretion of uric acid might play an important etiological role in Ca stone formation. Physicochemical studies indicate that if urate metabolism is so involved, the urate phase implicated must be monosodium urate.[9] The pK for the first proton of uric acid is 5.47.[12] Thus, in the urine of patients with urinary pH greater than 5.5 and an adequate sodium content, the monosodium urate is the stable phase (Figure 17). Moreover, in patients with hyperuricosuria, urine specimens are frequently supersaturated with respect to monosodium urate, principally because of high urate concentration in the urine (Figure 18).[9] Since these studies were performed following an adequate fluid intake (to achieve a urine volume of approximately 2 liters/day) and low sodium content (100 meq/day), a greater degree of supersaturation may have been anticipated in an uncontrolled customary setting. Unfortunately, the FPR (limit of metastability) of sodium urate in urine has not yet been measured. Nevertheless, the results indicate that monosodium urate could potentially form, in either a colloidal or a crystalline form, in the urine of patients with hyperuricosuric Ca urolithiasis.

Two hypotheses have been introduced to explain the formation of Ca stones in patients with hyperuricosuria. Each invokes an active participation of monosodium urate. In one scheme,[13] colloidal monosodium urate may form from urine supersaturated with respect to monosodium urate. Such a colloidal substance was believed to promote crystal aggregation of Ca oxalate, by adsorbing from urine certain inhibitors (acid mucopolysaccharide) of crystal aggregation. In support of this hypothesis, crystal aggregates of Ca oxalate were found to be more prominent in urine samples of high uric acid content.[14] Moreover, the inhibitor activity of acid mucopolysaccharide was found to be reduced in the presence of urate.[13] However, direct experimental verification for the removal of inhibitors by colloidal monosodium urate is lacking. Furthermore, it is

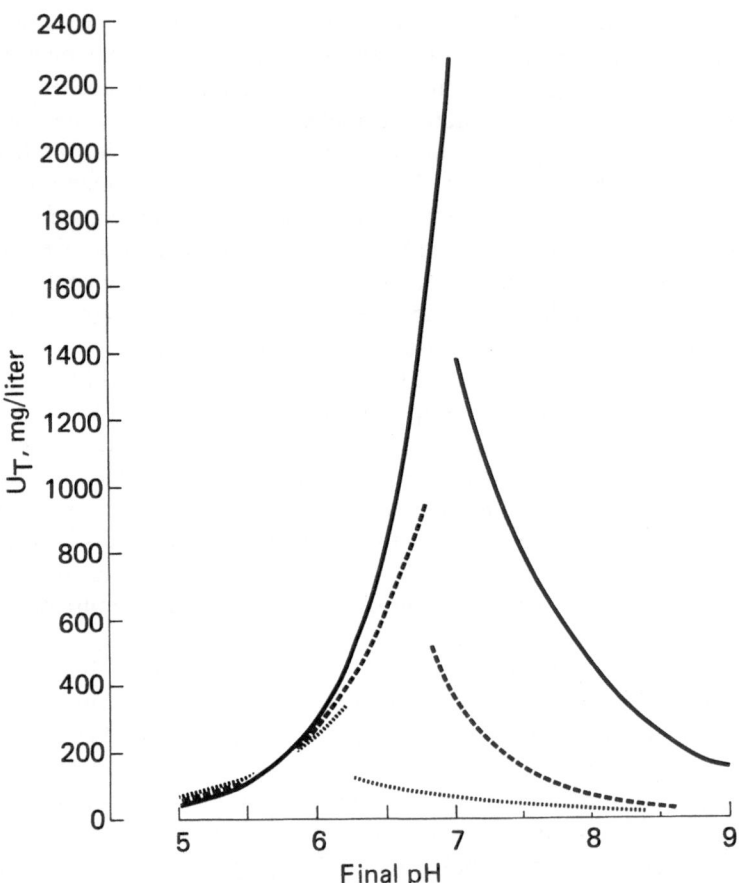

FIGURE 17. Uric acid solubility in the presence of sodium (Na). The concentrations of total dissolved urate (U_T) in the ambient solution after incubation of uric acid in 150 mM Na solution for varying periods at various pH are shown. The phase transition of uric acid to monosodium urate is indicated by a "break" in the solubility curve. [Na^+] equals 150 meq. (———) 2 hr; (– – –) 1 day; (......) 7 days.

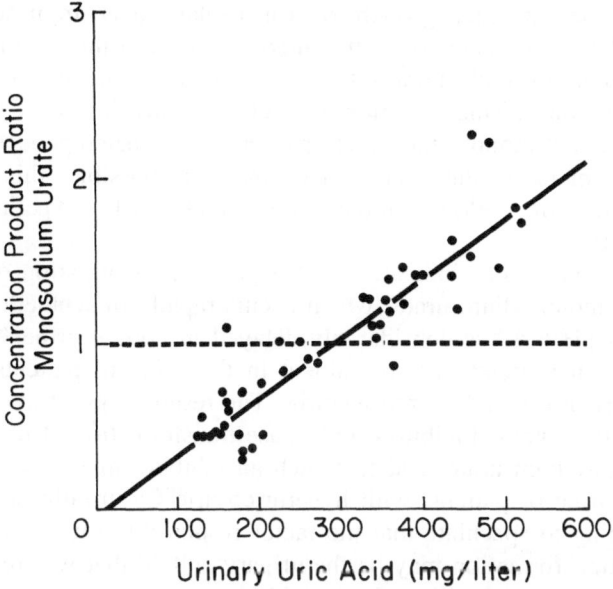

FIGURE 18. Dependence of concentration product ratio (state of saturation) of monosodium urate on the urinary concentration of uric acid. The horizontal dashed line indicates saturation with respect to monosodium urate. Points above this line indicate supersaturation; points below, undersaturation.

difficult to extrapolate to the nucleation of Ca oxalate in whole urine, since this study examined crystal aggregation (and growth) in diluted urine samples (1%). Nevertheless, this scheme is compatible with the infrequency with which crystalline monosodium urate is found in urine and in stones, since it does not require the crystallization of the urate salt.

An alternative hypothesis implicates an important role for crystalline monosodium urate, by invoking its involvement in heterogeneous nucleation of Ca salts.[15-17] As discussed in Chapter 2, solid seeds of monosodium urate are capable of inducing heterogeneous nucleation of Ca oxalate and Ca phosphate from solutions metastably supersaturated with respect to these Ca salts [see Figure 8 (Chapter 2)]. Crystalline axial arrangements have been shown to satisfy the epitaxial growth of Ca oxalate over monosodium urate.[18,19] The weakness of this theory resides in the finding that crystalline form of monosodium urate is infrequently found in urine or stones. This objection would be obviated if it were shown that colloidal monosodium urate participated in heterogeneous nucleation of Ca oxalate. Though theoretically possible, this mode of action for colloidal monosodium urate lacks experimental verification.

Recent studies indicate that the phase transformation of uric acid to monosodium urate, which occurs rapidly in synthetic solutions at pH 6.4,[9] is considerably delayed in normal urine.[20] This retardation is much less prominent in the urine of patients with hyperuricosuria and normocalciuria. The results suggest that urine normally contains inhibitor(s) of phase transformation of uric acid to monosodium urate, and that such an inhibitor may be deficient in the urine of patients with hyperuricosuric Ca urolithiasis. It is interesting to speculate that the factor responsible for the delayed phase transformation may be the urinary colloid that was reported to enhance the solubility of uric acid.[21]

CLINICAL PRESENTATION OF HYPERURICOSURIC CALCIUM UROLITHIASIS

Case 1. A 45-year-old white man had been passing renal stones since he was 35 years old. All stones were passed spontaneously. Analysis of stones disclosed the presence of Ca oxalate. He did not suffer from peptic ulcer disease, pathological skeletal fractures, gout, or recurrent urinary tract infection. He had no family history of nephrolithiasis or gout. A diet history disclosed an average daily consumption of two large servings of red meat or poultry, and 6 oz of wine.

The following tests were done and found to be normal: serum Ca, 9.6 mg%; serum P, 3.6 mg%; serum sodium, 140 meq/liter; potassium, 4.0 meq/liter; chloride, 102 meq/liter; carbon dioxide, 27 meq/liter; serum alkaline phosphatase activity, 80 IU; serum creatinine, 0.9 mg%; plasma glucose, 98 mg%; serum albumin, 4 g%; endogenous creatinine clearance, 102 ml/min; serum iPTH normal; 24-hour urinary cAMP, 4 μmol/g creatinine (normal); fasting urinary Ca,[22] 0.06 mg/mg creatinine (normal); urinary Ca following oral load of 1 g Ca,[22] 0.16 mg/mg creatinine (normal); 24-hr urinary Ca, 120–160 mg/day; urinary oxalate, 25 mg/day; qualitative urinary cystine, negative; urine culture, sterile.

Serum uric acid, however, was high normal at 6.8 mg%. Urinary uric acid, obtained once a week over a 3-week period on a random diet at home, was elevated (650–1100 mg/day). Urinary pH ranged from 5.8 to 6.5. Urine specimens were approximately twofold saturated with respect to monosodium urate.[9] When the patient was maintained on a low-purine diet, urinary uric acid gradually declined.

This case illustrates the typical presentation of hyperuricosuric Ca urolithiasis: (1) Ca urolithiasis, (2) persistent hyperuricosuria ($>$600 mg/day on a random diet), (3) urinary pH greater than 5.5, and (4) no abnormality of Ca metabolism, acid–base balance, or parathyroid function. Many cases may present a history of adherence to a high-purine diet; in these cases, hyperuricosuria may be ameliorated by a low-purine diet. Some cases may have a high endogenous production of uric acid. Allopurinol may be required to restore normal urinary uric acid. Clinical gout is uncommon. Men are more frequently affected than women.

The nature of stone disease in hyperuricosuric Ca urolithiasis may be indistinguishable from that of absorptive and renal hypercalciurias. The mean age of onset is between 30 and 40 years. It is uncommon in the first two decades of life. The disease tends to run a protracted course during the 3rd through 5th decades; it is usually of less severity after the 5th decade.[23]

It should be noted that hyperuricosuria may be associated with hypercalciurias.[6] In our experience, hyperuricosuria is encountered in approximately one third of cases with absorptive and renal hypercalciurias. The cause of the hyperuricosuria in hypercalciurias is probably the same as in hyperuricosuric Ca urolithiasis. When both hyperuricosuria and hypercalciuria occur in the same patient, the stone disease may be more severe than if only a single abnormality is present.

TREATMENT WITH ALLOPURINOL

In the majority of patients, hyperuricosuria may be corrected by a restriction of purine intake. However, because a low purine diet is difficult to maintain, allopurinol has generally been used.

Clinical Response. Several investigators have reported a favorable clinical response to allopurinol treatment (200–300 mg/day) in patients with Ca urolithiasis. In a controlled randomized study, Smith[11] found that patients on allopurinol therapy formed fewer Ca stones in comparison with those who received placebo. Coe and Raisen[8] found a significantly reduced stone episode during treatment when allopurinol alone was given to patients with hyperuricosuric Ca urolithiasis with normocalciuria, or when allopurinol was given with thiazide[24] in patients with hyperuricosuric Ca urolithiasis with hypercalciuria.

Physiological Action. Allopurinol, a xanthine oxidase inhibitor, impairs the synthesis of uric acid. It reduces serum and urinary uric acid in patients with either dietary hyperuricosuria or primary overproduction of uric acid. It does not influence parathyroid function or calcium metabolism, and does not alter renal excretion of calcium, orthophosphate, oxalate, magnesium, sodium, or potassium.[10] Urinary pH is also unaltered by therapy.[10] At high dosages (>400 mg/day), it may increase urinary pyrophosphate.[10]

Physicochemical Action. Allopurinol treatment reduces the urinary activity product ratio (APR) (state of saturation) of monosodium urate, principally by decreasing the urinary content of uric acid.[10] It does not alter the urinary APR of brushite or Ca oxalate.

Moreover, allopurinol therapy increases the urinary FPR[2] (limit of metastability) of Ca oxalate.[10] Its effect on the FPR of brushite is variable. There are two possible explanations for the increased FPR of Ca oxalate. First, the reduction in the APR of monosodium urate makes less likely the formation of colloidal or crystalline monosodium urate, and reduces the chance for the crystallization of Ca oxalate. Alternatively, allopurinol or its urinary metabolites may directly inhibit spontaneous nucleation of Ca oxalate.

FUTURE STUDIES

It is important to delineate more clearly the mechanism of Ca stone formation in patients with hyperuricosuria. The two proposed hypotheses, involving colloidal or crystalline monosodium urate, need to be better developed. Future efforts should include identification of colloidal or crystalline urate in urine, characterization of factors that regulate the phase transition of uric acid to monosodium urate, determination of the ability of colloidal urate to serve as heterologous seed, and direct demonstration of removal of inhibitors by urate. Since hyperuricosuria and hypercalciuria may both be present, the effects of combined therapy of allopurinol and thiazide or allopurinol and sodium cellulose phosphate should be determined from the standpoints of physical chemistry, physiological action, side effects, and clinical response.

REFERENCES

1. Pak, C. Y. C., Ohata, M., Lawrence, E. C., and Snyder, W. 1974. The hypercalciurias: Causes, parathyroid functions and diagnostic criteria. *J. Clin. Invest.* **54:**387–400.
2. Pak, C. Y. C., and Holt, K. 1976. Nucleation and growth of brushite and calcium oxalate in urine of stone-formers. *Metabolism* **25:**665–673.
3. Prien, E. L., and Prien, E. L., Jr. 1968. Composition and structure of urinary stone. *Am. J. Med.* **45:**654–672.
4. Gutman, A. B. 1968. Uric acid nephrolithiasis. *Am. J. Med.* **45:**756–779.
5. Henneman, P. H., Benedict, P. H., Forbes, A. P., and Dudley, H. R. 1958. Idiopathic hypercalciuria. *N. Engl. J. Med.* **259:**802–807.
6. Coe, F. L., and Kavalach, A. G. 1974. Hypercalciuria and hyperuricosuria in patients with calcium nephrolithiasis. *N. Engl. J. Med.* **291:**1344–1350.
7. Scott, J. T., Dixon, A. St. J., and Bywaters, E. G. L. 1964. Association of hyperuricaemia and gout with hyperparathyroidism. *Br. Med. J.* **1:**1070–1073.
8. Coe, F. L., and Raisen, L. 1973. Allopurinol treatment of uric-acid disorders in calcium-stone formers. *Lancet* **1:**129–131.
9. Pak, C. Y. C., Waters, O., Arnold, L., Holt, K., Cox, C., and Barilla, D. 1977. Mechanism for calcium urolithiasis among patients with hyperurico-

suria: Supersaturation of urine with respect to monosodium urate. *J. Clin. Invest.* **59**:426–431.

10. Barilla, D. E., and Pak, C. Y. C. 1977. In preparation.

11. Smith, M. J. V. 1977. Placebo vs. allopurinol for renal calculi. *J. Urol.* In press.

12. Finlayson, B., and Smith, A. 1974. Stability of first dissociable proton of uric acid. *J. Chem. Eng. Data* **19**:94–97.

13. Robertson, W. G. 1976. Physical chemical aspects of calcium stone-formation in the urinary tract. In *Urolithiasis Research.* H. Fleisch, W. G. Robertson, L. H. Smith, and W. Vahlensieck, Eds. Plenum Press, New York, pp. 25–39.

14. Robertson, W. G., Peacock, M., and Nordin, B. E. C. 1971. Calcium oxalate crystalluria and urine saturation in recurrent renal stone-formers. *Clin. Sci. (Oxford)* **40**:365–374.

15. Pak, C. Y. C., and Arnold, L. H. 1975. Heterogeneous nucleation of calcium oxalate by seeds of monosodium urate. *Proc. Soc. Exp. Biol. Med.* **149**:930–932.

16. Coe, F. L., Lawton, R. L., Goldstein, R. B., and Tembe, V. 1975. Sodium urate accelerates precipitation of calcium oxalate *in vitro. Proc. Soc. Exp. Biol. Med.* **149**:926–929.

17. Pak, C. Y. C., Hayashi, Y., and Arnold, L. H. 1976. Heterogeneous nucleation between urate, calcium phosphate and calcium oxalate. *Proc. Soc. Exp. Biol. Med.* **153**:83–87.

18. Lonsdale, K. 1968. Human stone. *Science* **159**:1159–1207.

19. Lonsdale, K. 1968. Epitaxy as a growth factor in urinary calculi and gallstones. *Nature (London)* **217**:56–58.

20. Zerwekh, J., and Pak, C. Y. C. 1977. In preparation.

21. Sperling, O., DeVries, A., and Kedem, O. 1965. Studies on the etiology of uric acid lithiasis. IV. Urinary non-dialyzable substances in idiopathic uric acid lithiasis. *J. Urol.* **94**:286–293.

22. Pak, C. Y. C., Kaplan, R. A., Bone, H., Townsend, J., and Waters, O. 1975. A simple test for the diagnosis of absorptive, resorptive and renal hypercalciurias. *N. Engl. J. Med.* **292**: 497–500.

23. Coe, F. L. 1977. Hyperuricosuric calcium oxalate nephrolithiasis. *Kidney Int.* Submitted for publication.

24. Coe, F. L. 1976. Long term prevention of calcium oxalate nephrolithiasis by chronic thiazide and allopurinol administration. *Clin. Res.* **24**:396A.

Chapter 6

Hyperoxaluric Calcium Urolithiasis

Hyperoxaluria may be either primary, consequent to an accelerated *in vivo* synthesis of oxalate, or secondary, associated particularly with certain gastrointestinal diseases. Since primary hyperoxaluria[1-4] is rare, this chapter will deal principally with the more common enteric hyperoxaluria.

HISTORICAL BACKGROUND

Ca urolithiasis has long been recognized as a complication of inflammatory diseases of the small bowel.[5,6] The cause of stone formation was believed to be related to the low urine output consequent to an excessive gastrointestinal fluid loss. More recently, however, several workers reported hyperoxaluria in certain diseases of the small bowel, and implicated it in the stone formation.

Hyperoxaluria has now been associated with Crohn's disease, ileal resection, or jejunoileal bypass surgery for morbid obesity.[7-13] The incidence of hyperoxaluria has been reported to be as high as 66%,[10] and that of stone (Ca oxalate) formation to be 25%.[14] Treatment with a large amount of Ca given orally (2–4 g Ca/day),[12] triglycerides,[12] or cholestyramine[9] has been reported to reduce renal oxalate excretion and ameliorate stone formation.

129

CAUSE OF THE HYPEROXALURIA

The underlying abnormality leading to hyperoxaluria in diseases of the small bowel was initially believed to be the result of a disturbed bile acid metabolism. One mechanism implicated the ileal malabsorption of glycine-conjugated bile salts.[15] The glycine moiety was then converted to glyoxylate by colonic bacterial action. Subsequent absorption and hepatic metabolism of glyoxylate to oxalate was considered to account for the hyperoxaluria. A second mechanism attributed the hyperoxaluria to the high hepatic synthesis of glycine and glyoxylate, as a result of increased bile acid turnover.[9] The third mechanism considered that there was a preferential hepatic synthesis of oxalate from glyoxylate.[7] This hypothesis could explain the normal renal excretion of glycolate despite hyperoxaluria, since increased excretion of both oxalate and glycolate would have been expected from the increased delivery of glyoxylate to the liver.

The mechanisms described above were later found to be inadequate.[10] The initial studies demonstrating that the administration of taurine could lower renal oxalate excretion, probably by impairing the formation of glycine-conjugated bile salts,[7,16] could not be confirmed.[17] Moreover, neither cholylglycine nor glyoxylate proved to be an important precursor of urinary oxalate in patients with ileal resections.[10]

It is now generally recognized that the hyperoxaluria in ileal disease is the result of an excessive intestinal absorption of oxalate.[10,11,13] The oxalate absorption has been measured from the recovery of oxalate radioactivity or the increase in urinary oxalate following an oral administration of either [^{14}C]oxalate or a stable oxalate load.[18] Since oxalate is not metabolized further *in vivo*,[19] and the kidney is the principal route of oxalate excretion, these techniques provide a reliable measure of oxalate absorption. A high intestinal absorption of oxalate has been demonstrated in ileal disease utilizing both methods.

The exact cause of the increased oxalate absorption has not been totally resolved. One theory implicates an increased availability of oxalate for absorption.[16] Under normal circumstances, much of dietary oxalate may be unavailable for absorption because of complexation by certain cations, particularly Ca and magnesium.[20] When there is malabsorption of fat, as is characteristic of ileal disease, the intraluminal content of Ca and magnesium may be reduced consequent to complexation of Ca and magnesium by fatty acids to form Ca or magnesium soaps. Thus, less divalent cations would be available to limit oxalate absorption. Oxalate absorption is increased because of an enlarged, free oxalate pool. Concurrently, intestinal absorption of Ca and magnesium might be expected to be reduced. This theory is supported by the following studies: (1) The degree of hyperoxaluria is positively correlated with the extent of fat malabsorption.[21] (2) Renal oxalate excretion is reduced by a low-fat diet or by substitution of a part of the dietary fat by medium-chain triglycerides.[12] (The latter maneuver reduces fecal fat and steatorrhea while maintaining caloric intake.) (3) Oral Ca or magnesium significantly reduces renal oxalate excretion.[12,18] (4) Oral sodium cellulose phosphate, which binds Ca and magnesium, increases the renal excretion of oxalate[22] (see Chapter 3).

This theory cannot account entirely for the increased oxalate excretion in ileal disease. Oral Ca or magnesium does not totally correct the hyperoxaluria,[18] although it usually decreases renal oxalate excretion. Moreover, the contention that urinary oxalate is positively correlated with fecal fat excretion has not been confirmed.[13] The results suggest that part of the increased oxalate excretion in ileal disease may occur independently of the action of intraluminal fatty acid or divalent cations

This conclusion is supported by the following observation: Following a stable oxalate load orally,[18] urinary oxalate increased within 2 hr, reaching a peak at 4 hr (Figure 19). The increase was much more prominent and sustained in patients with ileal disease than in control subjects, even when the oxalate load was given as soluble sodium oxalate, and after the role of intraluminal fatty acid or divalent cations was minimized by preparing patients on a diet low in oxalate and Ca and by fasting them for 12 hr prior to the oxalate loads. Preliminary data suggest that the high intestinal absorption in ileal disease may be the result of an increased perme-

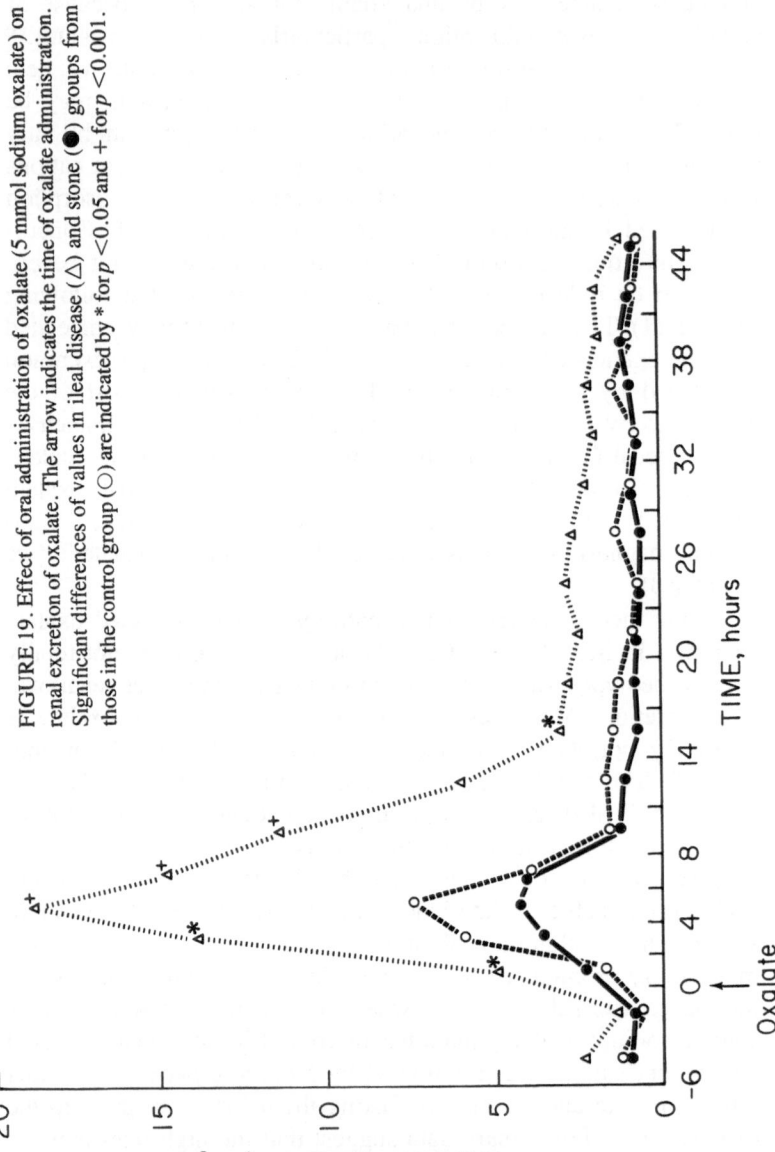

FIGURE 19. Effect of oral administration of oxalate (5 mmol sodium oxalate) on renal excretion of oxalate. The arrow indicates the time of oxalate administration. Significant differences of values in ileal disease (△) and stone (●) groups from those in the control group (○) are indicated by * for $p < 0.05$ and + for $p < 0.001$.

ability of the intestinal mucosa to oxalate from the action of bile salts or fatty acids.[23,24] This contention is supported by the finding that cholestyramine, which binds bile salts, may reduce renal oxalate excretion.[9] It is possible, however, that cholestyramine lowers urinary oxalate by directly binding oxalate in the intestinal tract.

In summary, the causes of the increased oxalate absorption in enteric hyperoxaluria is partly extrinsic (from the high "free" oxalate pool associated with steatorrhea) and partly intrinsic (from increased permeability to oxalate).

Site of Oxalate Absorption. Oxalate absorption is believed to occur as a passive process in all segments of the bowel.[25] Recent studies suggest that the colon is the site of and is required for the high oxalate absorption in enteric hyperoxaluria.[13] Hyperoxaluria is rarely encountered, and the intestinal oxalate absorption is normal in patients with steatorrhea in whom the colon is made "nonfunctional" by ileostomy. The proximal small bowel must also participate in oxalate absorption, however, since the increased renal oxalate excretion is encountered within 2 hr following an oral oxalate load in normal human subjects.[18]

It is not known whether the high colonic oxalate absorption in enteric hyperoxaluria is acquired from ileal disease or is intrinsic to that segment of the bowel. If oxalate absorption is intrinsically higher in the colon than in the small bowel, the high oxalate absorption and excretion in ileal disease could be partly explained by the shorter time period required for the oxalate load to enter the colon. Unfortunately, comparative studies of oxalate absorption in different parts of the bowel have not been conducted in normal human subjects or in patients with ileal disease.

CAUSE OF STONE FORMATION

The most important factor contributing to renal stone formation in ileal disease is probably the passage of urine supersaturated with respect to Ca oxalate. Because of hyperoxaluria and reduced urine volume, the urinary concentration of oxalate is markedly increased in patients with ileal disease who suffer from Ca oxalate urolithiasis. Thus, even though urinary Ca is usually low, urine specimens are often supersaturated with respect to Ca oxalate.[18] There is no evidence that renal excretion of inhibitors or promoters of nucleation is modified. The urinary FPR (limit of metastability) and rate of crystal growth of brushite and Ca oxalate are not significantly different from those of normal urine.

It is curious that Ca urolithiasis is present in a minority of patients with ileal disease, and that it is often absent even in the presence of marked hyperoxaluria. Some patients may have formed stones prior to the onset of ileal disease or may give a family history of nephrolithiasis. It has therefore been suggested that at least in some patients with secondary hyperoxaluria, there may have been other underlying abnormalities, which may have contributed to the renal stone formation.[26]

A factor that may protect patients with enteric hyperoxaluria from renal stone formation may be the reduced renal excretion of Ca associated with intestinal malabsorption of Ca. It should be noted that when urinary Ca is very low, urine specimens may not be excessively supersaturated with respect to Ca oxalate, despite hyperoxaluria.

CLINICAL PRESENTATION

The clinical presentation of enteric hyperoxaluria varies depending on the nature of the bowel disease. The onset of renal stone disease may be several months or years following the development of ileal disease. The disease may manifest as a large calculus in the renal pelvis, often requiring surgical removal, or as frequent passage of small calculi. The frequency of stone formation varies considerably, ranging from weekly to yearly. Stones are composed of Ca oxalate monohydrate or Ca oxalate dihydrate or both.

Typical biochemical presentations are (1) normal or low normal serum Ca and P, (2) low urinary Ca (<100 mg/day on a random diet), (3) high urinary oxalate (usually >60 mg/day), and (4) normal urinary glycolate and 1-glycerate. The normal renal excretion of glycolate and 1-glycerate distinguishes this condition from primary hyperoxaluria.[7] Urine volume may be low, when excessive gastrointestinal fluid loss is not compensated. Metabolic acidosis may be present consequent to bicarbonate loss in the feces; urinary pH is typically low, unlike the case in acidosis of renal origin. Parathyroid function may be stimulated because of the impairment in intestinal Ca absorption. Osteomalacia or osteoporosis may eventually develop.[27]

The total serum Ca concentration has been reported to be depressed in from 9 to 40% of patients with ileal disease in whom it was measured.[28,29] The significance of this observation is uncertain, since a large percentage of the patients also had hypoalbuminemia. The hypocalcemia is probably the consequence of several factors. First, intestinal Ca absorption may be significantly depressed in ileal disease.[30] Vitamin D deficiency, binding of Ca by unabsorbed fatty acids, and loss of mucosal surface (absorptive sites) probably contribute to the malabsorption of Ca. Second, hypomagnesemia, if it is present,[29,31] may cause hypocalcemia by inhibiting secretion[32] of or responsiveness[33] to PTH, or by impairing Ca–magnesium exchange in bone,[34,35] or both. Restoration of normal serum Ca concentration may be achieved by magnesium replacement therapy.

It should be recognized that while nephrolithiasis is rare in the presence of significant hypocalcemia (probably because of low urinary Ca), restoration of normocalcemia may invite development of renal stone disease.

Case 1. This 45-year-old lady taxi driver was well except for morbid obesity until 40 years of age, when she underwent jejunoileal bypass surgery. Prior to surgery, she had normal serum concentrations of Ca (9.5 mg%), P (3.6 mg%), and proteins. Over the ensuing 2 years, she experienced a substantial weight loss (277 to 130 lb). Approximately 6 months after surgery, however, she began to complain of carpopedal spasm, numbness in the fingertips, and twitching of the lips. By 1 year after surgery, these symptoms became so severe that she was unable to keep her job as a taxi driver.

At that time, she was found to have low serum Ca (7.7 mg%) and serum magnesium (1.0 mg%). Serum alkaline phosphatase activity and proteins were normal. Urinary Ca and magnesium were low at 16 and 7 mg/day, respectively. Urinary oxalate was high at 110 mg/day. The urinary activity product ratio[36] (APR) of Ca oxalate was 0.9; thus, urine specimens were undersaturated with respect to Ca oxalate, despite hyperoxaluria probably because of very low urinary Ca. No Ca oxalate crystals were found in fresh urine.

When the serum magnesium concentration was brought to the range of 1.7–1.9 mg% with intramuscular administration of magnesium, the serum concentration of Ca increased to 8.9–9.5 mg%, commensurate with considerable subjective improvement. Urinary Ca increased to 96 mg/day. She was discharged on oral magnesium (117 mg elemental magnesium as magnesium gluconate three times a day). On this medication, she continued to be free of symptoms of hypocalcemia and resumed her work as a taxi driver.

At 6 months after the initiation of magnesium therapy, however, she passed a renal stone of Ca oxalate. During the ensuing 3 years until the current admission, she had passed nearly 50 stones. Evaluation disclosed normal serum Ca of 9.8 mg% and magnesium of 2.0 mg%. Urinary Ca was 136 mg/day, and urinary oxalate was 82 mg/day. As compared with the results of initial evaluation (before magnesium replacement), urinary Ca increased nearly ninefold, while urinary oxalate decreased by only 25%. Thus, urine was 6.5-fold supersaturated with respect to Ca oxalate.

TREATMENT OF SECONDARY HYPEROXALURIA

This chapter will not consider the management of primary bowel disorder. The treatment of nephrolithiasis of secondary hyperoxaluria of ileal disease has been disappointing. Although several therapeutic modalities have been recommended, response to treatment has been variable and conflicting. Most of the approaches have been directed at reducing renal oxalate excretion. Limited data relevant to the physicochemical effects of drugs on stone formation, are available.

Oral Taurine. As discussed earlier, taurine was initially

shown to lower renal oxalate excretion.[7,16] Subsequent reports failed to document this finding.[17]

Cholestyramine. Oral administration of cholestyramine has been shown to reduce urinary oxalate.[9] By binding bile salts, cholestyramine may prevent the increased permeability of intestinal mucosa to oxalate produced by bile acids. Moreover, the drug may limit oxalate absorption by directly binding oxalate. However, these actions of cholestyramine may be counteracted by aggravation of steatorrhea, resulting from the smaller bile acid pool.

Oral Calcium or Magnesium. Oral Ca or magnesium has been shown to reduce renal oxalate excretion.[12,18] However, both divalent cations increase the renal excretion of Ca. Effects on the urinary APR (state of saturation) of Ca oxalate are variable. In some patients with ileal disease, oral Ca or magnesium may actually increase the urinary APR of Ca oxalate, and may be potentially harmful. As shown in the case report, oral magnesium therapy may cause stone formation *de novo.* Patients chosen for long-term treatment with Ca or magnesium should be those in whom the decrease in urinary oxalate during treatment is more prominent than the increase in urinary Ca.

Medium-Chain Triglycerides. Replacement of dietary fat by medium-chain triglycerides has been reported to lower urinary oxalate.[12] However, its effect on the urinary APR of Ca oxalate or on stone formation has not been quantitated.

General Recommendations. A rational recommendation for therapy of secondary hyperoxaluria of ileal disease is not currently possible, largely due to the limited knowledge regarding the mode of action of available drugs, and because of probable variable response to these drugs in different patients. The following general guidelines may be useful: (1) A low-oxalate diet should be instituted. Oxalate-rich foods, such as greens, spinach, asparagus, rhubarb, tea, citrus fruits, chocolate, and carrots, should be limited in the diet. Multivitamins may be given to avoid nutritional deficiency. Ingestion of large amounts of vitamin C should be avoided.[37] (2) Fluid intake should be sufficient to produce a urine output of at least 2 liters daily. (3) With any form of therapy, urinary Ca and oxalate should be carefully monitored.

FUTURE STUDIES

A better understanding of the cause of the enteric hyperoxaluria is needed. Application of the triple-lumen technique[38] promises to yield important information regarding the mechanism and site of oxalate absorption. This approach should determine whether hyperoxaluria is consequent to exclusion of Ca intraluminally or whether it is a manifestation of accelerated membrane transport of oxalate. From a diagnostic standpoint, candidates for jejunoileal bypass should be carefully screened.[39] Those with a propensity to form stones or with hypercalciuria, intestinal hyperabsorption of Ca, or a family history of stones should be excluded from surgery.

The area in which research is most needed is in the development of useful and effective treatment modalities. The physicochemical and physiological actions and side effects of currently available drugs should be better defined. New agents that inhibit intestinal oxalate absorption should be sought. A search for a nonabsorbable anionic-exchange resin with a high affinity for oxalate ion, for example, would seem warranted.

REFERENCES

1. Koch, J., Stokstad, E. L. R., Williams, H. E., and Smith, L. H., Jr. 1967. Deficiency of 2-oxo-glutarate:glyoxylate carboligase activity in primary hyperoxaluria. *Proc. Natl. Acad. Sci. U.S.A.* **57:**1123–1129.
2. Williams, H. E., and Smith, L. H., Jr. 1968. L-Glyceric aciduria. A new genetic variant of primary hyperoxaluria. *N. Engl. J. Med.* **278:**233–239.
3. Archer, H. E., Dormer, A. E. Scowen, E. F., and Watts, R. W. E. 1958. The aetiology of primary hyperoxaluria. *Br. Med. J.* **1:**175–181.
4. Solomons, C. C., Goodman, S. I., and Riley, C. M., 1967. Calcium carbimide in the treatment of primary hyperoxaluria. *N. Engl. J. Med.* **276:**207–210.
5. Gelzayd, E. A., Brewer, R. I., and Kirsner, J. B. 1968. Nephrolithiasis in inflammatory bowel disease. *Am. J. Dig. Dis.* **13:**1027–1034.
6. Maratka, A., and Nedbal, J. 1964. Urolithiasis as a complication of the surgical treatment of ulcerative colitis. *Gut* **5:**214–217.
7. Admirand, W. H., Earnest, D. L., and Williams, H. E. 1971. Hyperoxaluria and bowel disease. *Trans. Assoc. Am. Physicians* **84:**307–312.

8. Dowling, R. H., Rose, G. A., and Sutor, D. J. 1971. Hyperoxaluria and renal calculi in ileal disease. *Lancet* **1:**1103–1106.
9. Smith, L. H., Fromm, H., and Hofmann, A. F. 1972. Acquired hyperoxaluria, nephrolithiasis and intestinal disease: Description of a syndrome. *N. Engl. J. Med.* **286:**1371–1374.
10. Chadwick, V. S., Modha, K., and Dowling, R. H. 1973. Mechanism for hyperoxaluria in patients with ileal dysfunction. *N. Engl. J. Med.* **289:**172–176.
11. Stauffer, J. Q., Humphreys, M. H., and Weir, G. J. 1973. Acquired hyperoxaluria with regional enteritis after ileal resection: Role of dietary oxalate. *Ann. Intern. Med.* **79:**383–391.
12. Earnest, D. L., Williams, H. E. and Admirand, W. H. 1975. A physicochemical basis for treatment of enteric hyperoxaluria. *Trans. Assoc. Am. Physicians* **88:**224–234.
13. Dobbins, J. W., and Binder, H. J., 1977. Importance of the colon in enteric hyperoxaluria. *N. Engl. J. Med.* **296:**298–301.
14. Fikri, E., and Cassella, R. R. 1974. Jejunoileal bypass for massive obesity, results and complications in fifty-two patients, *Ann. Surg.* **179:**460–464.
15. Hofmann, A. F., Thomas, P. J., Smith, L. H., and McCall, J. T. 1970. Pathogenesis of secondary hyperoxaluria in patients with ileal resection and diarrhea. *Gastroenterology* **58:**960.
16. Dowling, R. H. 1973. Intestinal adaptation. *N. Engl. J. Med.* **288:**520–521.
17. Chadwick, V. S., and Modha, K. 1974. Hyperoxaluria with ileal dysfunction. *N. Engl. J. Med.* **290:**107–108.
18. Barilla, D. E., Notz, C., Kennedy, D., and Pak, C. Y. C. Renal oxalate excretion following oral oxalate loads in patients with ileal disease and with renal and absorptive hypercalciurias: Effect of calcium and magnesium. *Am. J. Med.* In press.
19. Edler, T. D., and Wyngaarden, J. B. 1960. The biosynthesis and turnover of oxalate in normal and hyperoxaluric subjects. *J. Clin. Invest.* **39:**1337–1344.
20. Archer, H. E., Dormer, A. E., Scowen, E. F., and Watts, R. W. E. 1957. Studies on the urinary excretion of oxalate by normal subjects. *Clin. Sci.* **16:**405–411.
21. Earnest, D. L., Johnson, G., Williams, H. E., and Admirand, W. H. 1974. Hyperoxaluria in patients with ileal resection: An abnormality in dietary oxalate absorption. *Gastroenterology* **66:**1114–1122.
22. Hayashi, Y., Kaplan, R. A., and Pak, C. Y. C. 1975. Effect of sodium cellulose phosphate therapy on crystallization of calcium oxalate in urine. *Metabolism* **24:**1273–1278.
23. Chadwick, V. S., Elias, E., Bell, G. D., *et al.* 1975. The role of bile acids in the increased intestinal absorption of oxalate after ileal resection. In *Advances in Bile Acid Research: IIIrd Bile Acid Meeting.* S. Matern, J. Hackenschmidt, and P. Back, Eds. F. K. Verlag, Stuttgart, pp. 435–440.

24. Dobbins, J. W., and Binder, H. J. 1976. Effect of bile salts and fatty acids on the colonic absorption of oxalate. *Gastroenterology* **70:**1096–1100.
25. Binder, H. J. 1974. Intestinal oxalate absorption. *Gastroenterology* **67:**441–446.
26. Gregory, J. 1976. Personal communication.
27. Pak, C. Y. C., and Fordtran, J. S. 1978. Disorders of mineral metabolism. In *Gastrointestinal Diseases,* 2nd ed. M. H. Schlesinger and J. S. Fordtran, Eds. W. B. Saunders, Philadelphia. In press.
28. Salmon, P. A. 1971. The results of small intestine bypass for the treatment of obesity. *Surg. Gynecol Obstet.* **132:**965–979.
29. Baddeley, M. 1973. Surgical treatment of obesity. *Proc. R. Soc. Med.* **66:**20–21.
30. Dano, P., and Christiansen, C. 1974. Calcium absorption and bone mineral contents following intestinal shunt operation in obesity: A comparison of three types of operations. *Scand. J. Gastroenterol.* **9:**775–779.
31. Swenson, S. A., Jr., Lewis, J. W., and Sebby, K. R. 1974. Magnesium metabolism in man with special reference to jejunoileal bypass for obesity. *Am. J. Surg.* **127:**250–255.
32. Suh, S. M. Csima, A., and Fraser, D. 1971. Pathogenesis of hypocalcemia in magnesium depletion: Normal end-organ responsiveness to parathyroid hormone. *J. Clin. Invest.* **50:**2668–2678.
33. Estep, H., Shaw, W. A., Watlington, C., Hobe, R., Holland, W., and Tucker, St.G. 1969. Hypocalcemia due to hypomagnesemia and reversible parathyroid hormone unresponsiveness. *J. Clin. Endocrinol.* **29:**842–848.
34. Chase, L. R., and Slatopolsky, E. 1974. Secretion and metabolic efficacy of parathyroid hormone in patients with severe hypomagnesemia. *J. Clin. Endocrinol. Metab.* **38:**363–381.
35. Pak, C. Y. C., and Diller, E. C. 1969. Ionic interaction with bone mineral. V. Effect of Mg^{2+}, $citrate^{3-}$, F^-, and SO_4^{2-} on the solubility, dissolution and growth of bone mineral. *Calcif. Tissue Res.* **4:**69–77.
36. Pak, C. Y. C., and Holt, K. 1976. Nucleation and growth of brushite and calcium oxalate in urine of stone-formers. *Metabolism* **25:**665–673.
37. Lamden, M. P., and Chrystowski, G. A. 1954. Urinary oxalate excretion by man following ascorbic acid ingestion. *Proc. Soc. Exp. Biol. Med.* **85:**190–192.
38. Brannan, P. G., Vergne-Marini, P., Pak, C. Y. C., Hull, A. R., and Fordtran, J. S. 1976. Magnesium absorption in the human small intestine: Patients with absorptive hypercalciuria. *J. Clin. Invest.* **57:**1412–1418.
39. Pak, C. Y. C., Kaplan, R. A., Bone, H., Townsend, J., and Waters, O. 1975. A simple test for the diagnosis of absorptive, resorptive and renal hypercalciurias. *N. Engl. J. Med.* **292:**497–500.

Chapter 7

Practical Guidelines for the Diagnosis and Management of Calcium Urolithiasis

While there has been a significant advancement in the urological management of patients with renal stones, many patients still undergo repeated urological procedures without examination of the cause of stone formation or a trial on a preventative medical regimen. In the light of recent advances in the understanding of the pathogenesis of nephrolithiasis, serious consideration should be given to the evaluation of patients with renal calculi in a search for the cause of urolithiasis. The value of such an evaluation derives from accumulating evidence that an appropriately selected treatment regimen may decrease the morbidity associated with this disease.[1,2]

As discussed in previous chapters, major progress has been made toward the development of reliable diagnostic criteria for the various causes of calcium urolithiasis. Unfortunately, many of the diagnostic procedures were developed in research centers, utilizing sophisticated procedures and a constant dietary regimen, and involving trained nursing, dietary, and technical personnel.[3] They may therefore be impractical, or may not have been tested for evaluation in an ambulatory setting.

This chapter summarizes the author's approach to the evaluation of ambulatory patients with calcium urolithiasis. It does not entail hospitalization. It requires three outpatient visits, and may be completed within a month. This evaluation depends largely on procedures that should be available in a routine clinical laboratory. Certain specialized procedures may be obtained commercially. The results of this evaluation correlate well with those of a more extensive assessment in an inpatient setting.[4] Moreover, the ambulatory evaluation provides certain information not available from inpatient examination—e.g., the influence of customary diet and habit on stone formation.

AMBULATORY EVALUATION

It is acknowledged that there may be other protocols that might be equally effective in providing discrimination among various causes of calcium urolithiasis. However, our protocol[4] will be described in detail in an effort to illustrate certain important aspects of diagnostic evaluation.

OUTLINE OF THE PROCEDURE (TABLE IX)

The patient may already have undergone urological evaluation (including abdominal roentgenogram or intravenous pyelogram and urine culture). If not, such an assessment is strongly recommended. If he recently had a urological procedure, e.g., pyelolithotomy, it is best to wait at least 3 weeks before initiating the study. A careful review of the treatment program should be made, and appropriate medications (e.g., thiazides, phosphates, or magnesium) should be withdrawn for 1 week preceding and throughout the period of evaluation.

(1) *First Visit.* When the patient is given an appointment for

TABLE IX. Outline of Ambulatory Protocol

Outline of procedures

Appointment day: Instruction on urine collection
Visit 1: History and physical examination
        24-hr urine on random diet
Visit 2: 24-hr urine on random diet
        Diet history and instruction
Visit 3: 24-hr urine on instructed diet (400 mg Ca, 100 meq Na/day)
        Fast and load

Outline of laboratory tests

				Urinary								
	CBC	SMA	PTH	Ca	UA	Cr	Na	pH	TV	Ox	cAMP	Qual. cystine urinalysis
Visit 1	X	X	X	X	X	X	X	X	X	X		X
Visit 2				X	X	X	X	X	X			
Visit 3		X		X	X	X	X	X	X		X	
Fast				X		X					X	
Load				X		X						

the first visit, he will be instructed to bring a 24-hr urine sample collected on a random diet. A simple instruction sheet, similar to the one presented in Table X, may be useful.

(a) *History and physical examination.* A careful "stone history" should be taken. We would recommend the use of a history outline as shown in Table XI. The extent and activity of stone disease may be ascertained from the number and frequency of stone passage or of urological procedures required for stones, particularly during the preceding 2 or 3 years. Stone composition, if available or known to the patient, may provide the diagnosis or suggest the area needing more thorough evaluation. The presence of struvite indicates infection with urea-splitting organisms.[5] Cystine stones are pathognomonic of cystinuria.[6] Urate stones suggest a disturbance in uric acid metabolism. Stones of Ca oxalate or Ca phosphate or both indicate disorders of oxalate or Ca metabolism.

TABLE X. How to Collect a 24-hr Urine Specimen at Home

Materials you will need

---

1. A clean plastic container with a screw-on lid.
2. A pitcher or can. Wash it out *thoroughly* and *dry* it before you use it.
3. Paper towel.
4. Ice chest or refrigerator.

Instructions for urine collection

Step 1. When you first get up in the morning, empty your bladder into the commode (just as you would normally do). (This urine sample is not to be saved.) Check what time it is.

Step 2. The next time you need to urinate, pass it either directly into the plastic container or into the pitcher or can. If you use the pitcher or can, go to Step 3. If you use the plastic container, go to Step 4.

Step 3. Carefully pour the urine from the pitcher or can into the container. Wipe the pitcher or can with the paper towel.

Step 4. Screw the lid onto the plastic container tightly and put the container into the refrigerator or ice chest.

Step 5. Repeat Steps 2–4 every time you urinate. On the following morning, get up at the same time (exactly 24 hours after beginning the urine collection). Pass urine and save it for the last time. Put the lid on *tightly* and return the container to the refrigerator or ice chest until it is time to bring it to the hospital.

Urine must be kept cold at all times.

A positive family history of stones suggests absorptive hypercalciuria, cystinuria, or primary hyperoxaluria. A history of peptic ulcer disease and pathologic skeletal fracture warrants a search for primary hyperparathyroidism.[7,8] Patients with gout may form stones of either uric acid or Ca oxalate. A history of chronic diarrhea, ileal disease, or intestinal surgery should arouse the suspicion of uric acid stones or Ca oxalate stones (enteric hyperoxaluria).[9] Absorptive hypercalciuria should be suspected in patients who are middle-aged Caucasian male, with a history of recurrent passage of calcium stones, with no history of bone disease, and who have a positive family history of renal stones. Renal hypercalciuria may be present in patients with a history of recurrent urinary tract infection.

A detailed history of dietary habits and drug ingestion should

TABLE XI. Stone History

Date: _____
Name: _____ Age: _____ Sex: _____ Race: _____
Occupation: _____
Onset: _____
No. spontaneously passed: Total: _____ Last 3 years: _____
Surgical removal: _____
Structural abnormality of urinary tract? _____
Stone analysis: _____ Radiopaque? _____
Family history of stones: _____
Intestinal disease, resection: _____ Chronic diarrhea: _____
Peptic ulcer: _____ Skel. fracture: _____ Gout: _____ Urinary tract infection: _____
Lab. test: High serum Ca? _____ High urine Ca? _____ High serum uric acid? _____
   High urin. uric acid? _____ Other? _____
Diet hx: Tea: _____ Milk: _____ Dairy products: _____
   Fluid intake: _____
Treatment: Phosphates? _____ Mg: _____
   Thiazides? _____ Zyloprim? _____
Medications: Antacids? _____ Vitamin C? _____
   Vitamin D? _____ Calcium? _____
   Other: _____
Existing stones? _____
Other disorders: _____

---

be taken. A high-Ca diet, as from an ingestion of an excessive amount of dairy products, may aggravate the stone disease in those patients with an intestinal hyperabsorption of Ca. A high-purine diet may cause hyperuricosuria and Ca stone formation (hyperuricosuric calcium urolithiasis).[10] Adrenocorticosteroids, nonabsorbable antacids that bind phosphate, and vitamin D (in pharmacological amounts) may cause hypercalciuria. Vitamin C and ingestion of oxalate-rich foods (e.g., tea, chocolate) in excessive amounts may increase renal oxalate excretion.[11] Acetazolamide may cause Ca phosphate urolithiasis by impairing renal acidification. Xanthine stones may develop, though rarely, during allopurinol therapy.[12]

Unfortunately, the physical examination rarely yields any specific diagnostic clues. Band keratopathy suggests chronic hypercalcemia or a high circulating $Ca \times P$ product, or both. The presence of tophi indicates gout and associated stones. Adenopathy or hepatosplenomegaly suggests a myeloproliferative syndrome and uric acid stones.

(*b*) *Laboratory tests*. The stone analysis should be determined, if it was not previously done and if the stone is available. It may be obtained from several commercial laboratories, including Urolithiasis Laboratory, P.O. Box 25375, Houston, Texas, and Louis C. Herring and Co., P.O. Box 2191, Orlando, Florida. A urological roentgenogram should be obtained, if it has not been performed previously. Uric acid and xanthine stones are radiolucent. Ca-containing stones and stones of struvite and cystine are radiopaque. Staghorn calculi may be seen with urinary tract infection, cystinuria, or primary hyperparathyroidism. Nephrocalcinosis may be encountered in renal tubular acidosis, primary hyperparathyroidism, or chronic pyelonephritis. It should be distinguished from medullary sponge kidney, which may coexist with primary hyperparathyroidism or hypercalciuria.[13,14]

On the first visit (see Table IX), blood studies (on fasting venous blood) comprise complete peripheral blood cell count (CBC); a multichannel screen (SMA) including serum Ca, P, total proteins, albumin, alkaline phosphatase, sodium, potassium, carbon dioxide, chloride, creatinine, and uric acid; and serum immunoreactive parathyroid hormone (iPTH). Urine tests include spot sample for urinalysis and qualitative cystine, and 24-hr sample for Ca, uric acid (UA), creatinine (Cr), sodium, pH, total volume (TV), and oxalate (Ox). Serum iPTH and urinary oxalate may be obtained commercially (e.g. from Mayo Medical Laboratories, Rochester, Minn. and Bio-Science Laboratories, Van Nuys, California).

(2) *Second Visit*. Another 24-hr urine sample collected on a random diet is to be analyzed for Ca, uric acid, creatinine, sodium, pH, and total volume. Diet history is to be taken, and the patient is instructed on a diet of approximately 400 mg Ca and 100 meq sodium/day, to be maintained until the third visit (at least 1 week). The diet instruction presented in Table XII may be useful. (At this juncture, this diet is intended for diagnostic purposes only; it is not meant for treatment.)

TABLE XII. Limited Calcium–Limited Sodium Diet

This diet limits calcium and sodium. Certain foods that have large amounts of oxalate or purine are also limited. Foods containing these substances do not cause formation of kidney stones, but if they are taken in large amounts, they can add to the problem. If you follow this diet closely, we will be able to see the degree to which diet may influence kidney stone formation.

Food group	Foods allowed	Foods not allowed
Beverages	Carbonated drinks; coffee; lemonade, limeade; decaffeinated coffee	ALL MILK including canned milk, eggnog, milk shakes, malted milk, powdered milk, and buttermilk; hot chocolate, cocoa mixes; tea; alcoholic beverages
Bread and cereals	Biscuits, bread, buns (hamburger), corn bread, muffins, pancakes, sweet rolls, flour tortillas, waffles; cooked and dry cereals	Salt-topped bread, crackers, and rolls; corn tortillas; vitamin-supplemented cereals.
Cheese	None	ALL CHEESE including cheddar cheese, cheese crackers, cheese foods, cheese puffs, cheese sauces, cheese sticks, cheese spreads, cottage cheese, cream cheese, dips, Gouda, Parmesan, processed cheese, provolone, Romano, and Swiss cheese.
Desserts and sweets	Honey, jelly, jam, marmalade, preserves, syrup, sugar; fruit cobblers, fruit pies; gelatin desserts; white and yellow cake with sugar icing, shortcake; bread pudding (no milk), tapioca; lemon sauce made with cornstarch; cookies, vanilla wafers, graham crackers; fruit ices and popsicles	Molasses; chiffon pie, cream pie; ALL CHOCOLATE in cakes, icings, pies and cookies, chocolate chips, and chocolate syrup; pudding, custard; Boston cream pie; rice pudding; yogurt; ALL ICE CREAM, mellorine, frozen custard, ice milk, sherbet, and "dietetic" ice cream

(Continued)

TABLE XII. (*Continued*)

Food group	Foods allowed	Foods not allowed
Fats	Butter, margarine, vegetable oil, and most salad dressings; powdered or liquid nondairy creamer; nondairy whipped topping	Salad dressings made with cheese or sour cream; cream, half-and-half
Fruits and juices	Fresh, canned, and frozen fruit; fresh, canned, and frozen fruit juice	Dried fruits; tomato juice and vegetable juice cocktail; powdered fruit juice substitutes
Meats and meat substitutes	Eggs TWO AVERAGE PORTIONS PER DAY of baked, boiled, broiled, or fried beef, chicken, freshwater fish, fresh pork, seafood, tuna, turkey, veal or venison; homemade chili, meat pies and stews	ALL ORGAN MEATS—liver, brains, etc. Barbequed, cured, salty or smoked meat and fish; ALL bacon, anchovies, canned meat and stews, canned salmon, caviar, canned chili, corned beef, corned beef hash, dried chipped beef; ALL frankfurters, ham, herring; ALL luncheon meats, frozen meat pies, pizza, salt pork, sardines, tamales; ALL sausage, T.V. dinners, and textured vegetable protein (soybean) breakfast products
Starches	Corn, macaroni, noodles, potatoes, rice, and spaghetti; dried beans and dried peas in moderation	Macaroni and cheese; potato chips, corn chips, tortilla chips; corn pudding
Vegetables and soups	Fresh, canned, and frozen vegetables; homemade soups	Sauerkraut and other vegetables prepared in brine; canned pork and beans; hominy; ALL "GREENS" such as turnip greens, spinach, collard greens, mustard greens, beet greens, and polk; Chinese vegetables; ALL CANNED SOUP, cheese soups, canned broth, bouillon cubes

Miscellaneous	Spices, herbs, and extracts; unsalted peanut butter; SMALL AMOUNTS OF meat tenderizer, brown gravy, and sauces such as catsup, chili sauce, spaghetti sauce, steak sauce, and Worcestershire sauce because these DO CONTAIN SALT!	ADDED SALT, seasoned salt, monosodium glutamate (MSG), and salt substitutes; artificial sweeteners; prepared horseradish and mustard; olives, pickles, salted nuts, salted popcorn; regular peanut butter; soy sauce; cream gravies and white sauce, hollandaise, newburg sauce
Supplements	None	Amino acid or protein supplements; multivitamins, vitamins plus iron, vitamins plus minerals, and VITAMIN C
Medications	As directed by physician	Aspirin, sodium bicarbonate; antacids and milk of magnesia

Instructions for limiting salt:

1. Use no salt or seasoned salt at the table.
2. Eat foods only lightly salted during preparation.
3. Do not add salt in the preparation of foods to which salt is added in processing. Example: canned vegetables.
4. When preparing food from a recipe, use half the amount of salt specified.

(3) *Third Visit.* The 24-hr urine sample collected on the instructed diet is to be assayed for Ca, uric acid, creatinine, sodium, pH, total volume, and cyclic AMP (cAMP) (which may be obtained commercially, e.g., from Bio-Science Laboratories or Bio-Assay Laboratory, P.O. Box 6113, Dallas, Texas). Fasting venous blood is to be analyzed again for SMA.

During this visit, patients undergo studies of "fast and load." [15] Following a 12-hr fast (from the previous suppertime) except for distilled water, a 2-hr fasting urine sample is to be obtained and analyzed for Ca, creatinine, and cAMP. Patients then ingest a liquid synthetic meal (Doyle Pharmaceutical Co., Minneapolis, Minnesota) containing 1 g Ca. A urine sample collected over the subsequent 4 hr is to be assayed for Ca and creatinine. The simple instruction shown in Table XIII may be helpful. It should be emphasized that the value of fasting urinary Ca depends on the preparation of patients on a low-Ca–low-Na diet prior to the test. In patients with intestinal hyperabsorption of Ca, "abnormally" high values of fasting urinary Ca may be found if they were not so prepared.

TABLE XIII. Instructions to Patient for "Fast and Load" Test

For at least 1 week prior to the test, adhere to a low-calcium, low-sodium diet.

Day before test: Date:_____

1. Drink 10 oz (300 ml) of distilled water at *7 p.m.*
2. Drink 10 oz (300 ml) of distilled water at *midnight.*
3. Fast from *7 p.m.* except for water.

Day of test: Date:_____

4. At *7 a.m.*, empty bladder and discard urine.
   Drink 20 oz (600 ml) of distilled water.
5. From *7 a.m.* to *9 a.m.* (for 2 hours), collect all urine.
   Keep cold.
6. Bring urine collection to _____.
   Be there at *9 a.m.*
7. At *9 a.m.*, you will receive a liquid food containing calcium.
   You will be collecting urine for 4 hours 'til *1 p.m.*
   You will be drinking 10 oz (300 ml) of distilled water at *11 a.m.*

INTERPRETATION OF DATA

Hypercalciurias. Hypercalciuria may be defined as urinary Ca exceeding 200 mg/day on a diet restricted in Ca and sodium (third urine sample). Values above this limit have been shown to correlate well with urinary supersaturation with respect to brushite and Ca oxalate.[16] Urinary Ca on a random diet (first two urine samples) is typically higher than on a restricted diet. Greater intake of Ca and sodium probably contribute to this augmented Ca excretion.

Hyperuricosuric Calcium Urolithiasis. The upper range of normal for uric acid in our laboratory is 600 mg/day, which is lower than in other laboratories. Hyperuricosuria defined by this limit has been found to correlate well with the urinary supersaturation with respect to monosodium urate[17] and with the propensity for Ca stone formation. In patients with hyperuricosuric Ca urolithiasis, urinary uric acid is greater than 600 mg/day in two, or in all three, specimens. Urinary pH is greater than 5.5. Hypercalciuria may coexist with hyperuricosuria.

Hyperoxaluria. Significant hyperoxaluria (urinary oxalate >80 mg/day) indicates that primary[18] or enteric hyperoxaluria[9] is probably present. A mild to moderate hyperoxaluria (urinary oxalate 40–80 mg/day) may occur with vitamin C therapy,[11] overindulgence with oxalate-rich foods, or severe dietary Ca deprivation.[19]

In enteric hyperoxaluria, low values for urinary Ca, serum Ca, magnesium, and carbon dioxide may be found.

Uric Acid Stones. Typically, urinary pH is unusually low (<5.5) and serum uric acid high. Urinary uric acid may be normal or high. A microscopic examination of urinary sediment may show the presence of uric acid crystals.

Renal Tubular Acidosis.[20] This condition may be suggested by high urinary pH (6.7–7.3), low serum carbon dioxide concentration, hyperchloridemia, and hypokalemia. Nephrocalcinosis is more common than nephrolithiasis. Endogenous creatinine clearance and urinary Ca may be reduced.

Cystinuria.[6] If qualitative urinary cystine is positive, a more extensive evaluation, including quantitative measurement of cystine excretion, is recommended.

Infection Stones.[5] Pyuria, positive urine culture for urea-splitting organisms, and high urinary pH (>7) suggest that the potential for the formation of struvite stones is present.

Diagnostic criteria for different causes of hypercalciuria are presented in Table III (Chapter 3). Table XIV, which may be used to tabulate urinary data, presents normal ranges for our laboratory.

OPTIMUM TREATMENT OF CALCIUM UROLITHIASIS

The current status of clinical efficacy studies for the treatment of Ca urolithiasis is disappointing. The problem is twofold: (1) the widespread practice of random therapy in which treatment is provided irrespective of the cause of the disease and without clear indications and (2) the inherent difficulty in conducting a good pharmacological efficacy study in urolithiasis.

Sufficient progress has been made in urolithiasis research to allow formulation of criteria for optimum therapy whereby a specific treatment is provided for each cause of urolithiasis, depending on its ability to "correct" the underlying disorder and "reverse" the physicochemical abnormality in the urine.[1] The following optimum criteria are admittedly tentative, and will need to be continually revised, pending future findings in urolithiasis research. It is assumed that optimum therapy may be made more effective in preventing stone formation and may be associated with less complications than a random therapy.

Primary Hyperparathyroidism. Parathyroidectomy.

Absorptive Hypercalciuria Type I. Sodium cellulose phosphate, 5 g two or three times a day orally with meals[1]; a low-Ca diet (avoidance of dairy products); magnesium gluconate, 1–1.5 g twice a day separately from sodium cellulose phosphate (to avoid magnesium depletion). If ineffective or poorly tolerated, thiazide as in renal hypercalciuria.

Absorptive Hypercalciuria Type II. Instruction on a low-Ca diet. If ineffective, sodium cellulose phosphate as in absorptive hypercalciuria Type I.

TABLE XIV. Urinary Data

Patient:_____

	Normal range	Day 1 (Random diet) Date	Day 2	Day 3 (400 mg Ca/d)	Fast (12 hr)	Ca load (1 g p.o.)
Routine urinalysis						
Protein						
Glucose						
WBC						
RBC						
Crystalluria						
24-hr samples						
TV (ml/d)						
pH						
Ca (mg/d)	<200					
Na (meq/d)						
Uric acid (mg/d)	<600					
Oxalate (mg/d)	<40					
cAMP (μmol/gCr)	<5.4					
Cystine, qualitative						
Fast						
Ca/Cr (mg/mg)	<0.11					
cAMP (μmol/g Cr)	<6.85					
Load						
Ca/Cr (mg/mg)	<0.20					
Endog Cr Cl[a] (ml/min)	>90					

[a] Endogenous creatinine clearance.

Absorptive Hypercalciuria Type III (*with Hypophosphatemia*). Orthophosphate,[21] 500 mg P three or four times a day orally. Commercial preparations include K-Phos and NeutraPhos.

Renal Hypercalciuria. Thiazide[22] (hydrochlorothiazide, 50 mg twice a day; trichloromethiazide, 4 mg a day; or chlorthalidone, 50 mg a day), with potassium supplements (40–60 meq in divided doses each day) if necessary.

Absorptive Hypercalciuria with Hyperuricosuria. Add allopurinol, 100 mg three times a day.

Renal Hypercalciuria with Hyperuricosuria. Add allopurinol, 100 mg three times a day.

Hyperuricosuric Calcuim Urolithiasis.[2] Allopurinol, 100 mg three times a day, and avoidance of excess sodium intake.

In all cases, fluid intake sufficient to achieve urine output of at least 2 liters per day is strongly recommended.

FOLLOW-UP CARE

Subsequent to initiation of treatment, patients should be followed at regular intervals. Such follow-up care is intended to (1) assure safety of treatment, (2) assess therapeutic efficacy, (3) allow initiation of an improved or alternate treatment regimen, and (4) provide an opportunity for temporary cessation of therapy.

It is our customary practice to give patients appointments on an ambulatory basis at 1 month after initiaton of treatment, and at 4- to 6-month intervals thereafter. Tests ordered at these visits depend on the specific hazards and requirements of the particular treatment regimen. The importance of adhering to the prescribed regimen and of maintaining high urine output should be emphasized at each visit.

After 1–2 years of treatment, therapy may be stopped temporarily when it is considered successful. If biochemical abnormalities persist, the treatment may be resumed. If they are no longer present, therapy may be withheld. This program therefore allows delivery of care only when the need is present.

SELECTION OF PATIENTS FOR EVALUATION
AND TREATMENT

In the patient who is actively forming many stones, diagnostic evaluation and treatment are clearly indicated.

The disposition of the patient who has formed just one stone is more difficult. It is our conviction that anyone who has recently formed a stone should be evaluated for the cause of stone formation, unless a remediable cause (e.g., acetazolamide therapy) has been identified. The cost of evaluation is small, when considered in the context of the expense of hospitalization and morbidity that may ensue from a potential new stone formation. If the underlying cause is discovered, we recommend that the patient be treated according to the regimen described previously, even though he may have formed only one stone. This recommendation assumes that certain biochemical abnormalities (e.g., hypercalciuria, hyperuricosuria, and hyperoxaluria) may be pathogenetically important in stone formation, that the correction of such abnormalities may prevent new stone formation, and that the rate of recurrence is high.

REFERENCES

1. Pak, C. Y. C., Delea, C. S., and Bartter, F. C. 1974. Successful treatment of recurrent nephrolithiasis (calcium stones) with cellulose phosphate. *N. Engl. J. Med.* **290:**175–180.
2. Coe, F. L., and Raisen, L. 1973. Allopurinol treatment of uric acid disorders in calcium-stone formers. *Lancet* **1:**129–131.
3. Pak, C. Y. C., Ohata, M., Lawrence, E. C., and Snyder, W. 1974. The hypercalciurias: Causes, parathyroid functions and diagnostic criteria. *J. Clin. Invest.* **54:**387–400.
4. Pak, C. Y. C., Fetner, C., Townsend, J., Brinkley, L., Northcutt, C., Barilla, D. E., Kadesky, M., and Peters, P. 1977. Ambulatory evaluation of calcium urolithiasis: Comparison of results with those of inpatient evaluation. *Am. J. Med.* In press.
5. Griffith, D. P., and Musher, D. M. 1973. Prevention of infected urinary stones by urease inhibition. *Invest. Urol.* **11:**228–233.
6. Bartter, F. C., Lotz, M., Thier, S., Rosenberg, L. E., and Potts, J. T., Jr. 1965. Cystinuria: Combined clinical staff conference at the National Institutes of Health. *Ann. Intern. Med.* **62:**796–822.
7. Kaplan, R. A., Snyder, W. H., Stewart, A., and Pak, C. Y. C. 1976. Metabolic effects of parathyroidectomy in asymptomatic primary hyperparathyroidism. *J. Clin. Endocrinol. Metab.* **42:**415–426.
8. Bone, H. G., III, Snyder, W. H., and Pak, C. Y. C. 1977. Diagnosis of hyperparathyroidism. *Annu. Rev. Med.* **28:**111–117.
9. Earnest, D. L., Williams, H. E., and Admirand, W. H. 1975. A physicochemical basis for treatment of enteric hyperoxaluria. *Trans. Assoc. Amer. Physicians* **88:**224–234.
10. Coe, F. L., and Kavalach, A. G. 1974. Hypercalciuria and hyperuricosuria in patients with calcium nephrolithiasis. *N. Engl. J. Med.* **291:**1344–1350.
11. Lamden, M. P., and Chrystowski, G. A. 1954. Urinary oxalate excretion by man following ascorbic acid ingestion. *Proc. Soc. Exp. Biol. Med.* **85:**190–192.
12. Seegmiller, J. E. 1968. Xanthine stone formation. *Am. J. Med.* **45:**780–783.

13. Rao, D. S., Frame, B., Block, M. A., and Parfitt, A. M. 1977. Primary hyperparathyroidism: A cause of hypercalciuria and renal stones in patients with medullary sponge kidney. *J. Am. Med. Assoc.* **237:**1353–1355.

14. Gremillion, D. H., Kee, J. W., and McIntosh, D. A. 1977. Hyperparathyroidism and medullary sponge kidney: A chance relationship? *J. Am. Med. Assoc.* **237:**799–800.

15. Pak, C. Y. C., Kaplan, R. A., Bone, H., Townsend, J., and Waters, O. 1975. A simple test for the diagnosis of absorptive, resorptive, and renal hypercalciurias. *N. Engl. J. Med.* **292:**497–500.

16. Pak, C. Y. C., and Holt, K. 1976. Nucleation and growth of brushite and calcium oxalate in urine of stone-formers. *Metabolism* **25:**665–673.

17. Pak, C. Y. C., Waters, O., Arnold, L., Holt, K., Cox, C., and Barilla, D. 1977. Mechanism for calcium urolithiasis among patients with hyperuricosuria: Supersaturation of urine with respect to monosodium urate. *J. Clin. Invest.* **59:**426–431.

18. Williams, H. E., and Smith, L. H., Jr. 1968. L-Glyceric aciduria: A new genetic variant of primary hyperoxaluria. *N. Engl. J. Med.* **278:**233–239.

19. Hayashi, Y., Kaplan, R. A., and Pak, C. Y. C. 1975. Effect of sodium cellulose phosphate therapy on crystallization of calcium oxalate in urine. *Metabolism* **24:**1273–1278.

20. Morris, R. C., Jr. 1969. Renal tubular acidosis: Mechanisms, classification and implications. *N. Engl. J. Med.* **281:**1405–1413.

21. Smith, L. H., Thomas, W. C., Jr., and Arnaud, C. D. 1973. Orthophosphate therapy in calcium renal lithiasis. In *Urinary Calculi: Proceedings of the International Symposium on Renal Stone Research, Madrid, 1972.* L. C. Delatte, A. Rapado, and A. Hodgkinson, Eds. Karger, Basel and New York, pp. 188–197.

22. Coe, F. L., Canterbury, J. M., Firpo, J. J., and Reiss, E. 1973. Evidence for secondary hyperparathyroidism in idiopathic hypercalciuria. *J. Clin. Invest.* **52:**134–142.

Index

157